A QUESTION OF LIFE

The Warnock Report on
Human Fertilisation and Embryology

Mary Warnock

Basil Blackwell

© Crown copyright 1984. Reprinted by permission of the
   Controller of Her Majesty's Stationery Office.
© Additional material (Introduction and Conclusion) Mary Warnock 1985

First published 1985

Basil Blackwell Ltd
108 Cowley Road, Oxford OX4 1JF, UK

Basil Blackwell Inc.
432 Park Avenue South, Suite 1505,
New York, NY 10016, USA

British Library Cataloguing in Publication Data
Great Britain. *Committee of Inquiry into Human Fertilisation and Embryology*
   The Warnock report: report of the Committee of Inquiry into Human
   Fertilisation and Embryology.
   1. Infertility—Treatment—Social aspects
   I. Title   II. Warnock, Mary
   363.9'6   RC889

   ISBN 0-631-14257-6

Library of Congress Cataloging in Publication Data applied for

Additional material typeset by Katerprint Co. Ltd, Oxford
Printed in Great Britain by Whitstable Litho, Whitstable, Kent

CONTENTS

MEMBERS OF THE COMMITTEE

Dr A McLaren MA DPhil FRS	Director, Medical Research Council Mammalian Development Unit.
Mr D J McNeil WS	Solicitor, Edinburgh.
Professor K Rawnsley CBE MB ChB FRCPsych FRCP DPM	Professor of Psychological Medicine, Welsh National School of Medicine.
Mrs M J Walker JP MA APSW	Psychiatric social worker, former student counsellor at Cambridge University.

Joint Secretaries
Mrs J C Croft
Dr J S Metters

Legal Adviser
Mr R A Sanders

Observers
Dr M Hennigan, Scottish Home and Health Department
Mr L Webb, Department of Education and Science.

LETTER FROM MARY WARNOCK TO THE GOVERNMENT

The Rt Hon Norman Fowler	Secretary of State for Social Services.
The Lord Hailsham PC	Lord Chancellor.
The Rt Hon Sir Keith Joseph	Secretary of State for Education and Science.
The Rt Hon George Younger	Secretary of State for Scotland.
The Rt Hon Nicholas Edwards	Secretary of State for Wales.
The Rt Hon James Prior	Secretary of State for Northern Ireland.

Sirs

I have the honour to present the report of the Committee of Inquiry into Human Fertilisation and Embryology established in July 1982 to examine the social, ethical and legal implications of recent, and potential developments in the field of human assisted reproduction.

The task you set the Inquiry was not an easy one. The issues raised reflect fundamental moral, and often religious, questions which have taxed philosophers and others down the ages. Rightly you chose a membership which encompassed not only the many professions with a concern in these matters but the many religious traditions within society, so that as many viewpoints as possible could be brought to bear on the morally sensitive issues before us. I would like to take this opportunity to place on record my gratitude to all the members of the Inquiry for their hard work, their enthusiasm and commitment, and more especially for the way they have brought their own values to the consideration of the problems before us and yet at the same time have been open and responsive to the attitudes and beliefs of others. I am also grateful for the way in which we have been able to share our professional expertise, a process which I am sure has enhanced the report, by helping us to see the problems in a broader perspective.

Despite the way in which members have worked together, there remain nonetheless certain differences between us; indeed it would have been surprising if, on such sensitive issues, we had been united. These differences, presented in three formal expressions of dissent have, significantly, focussed on the very subjects, surrogacy and research on human embryos, which, to judge from the evidence, arouse the greatest public anxiety. Thus even in our disagreement we have reflected the range of views within society.

It is not possible that a report like this should be equally well received in all quarters, given some of the controversial issues we have had to consider. There is bound to be criticism that we have gone too far, or not far enough. However, we have sought to provide on the one hand a reasoned discussion of the issues which we hope will contribute to a high standard of public debate on matters which are of deep concern to the public, and on the other a coherent set of proposals for how public policy, rather than the individual conscience, should respond to a range of developments which many people will not wish to participate in, but which others find entirely acceptable. We have tried in short, to give due consideration both to public and to private morality.

Finally, I would like to add my thanks to those members of the Department who have helped us to produce our report. We have benefitted greatly from the advice of Mr R A Sanders on the legal aspects of our work, and his help has been indispensable. But our most grateful thanks must go to our joint secretaries, Mrs J C Croft and Dr J S Metters whose patience, humour and unflagging energy have been beyond praise. We could not have been better served.

Mary Warnock
26 June 1984

INTRODUCTION

The Times, on 15 December 1984, carried a dramatic headline. It read "Warnock: Ethics Undermined". What followed was a denunciation of the Report of the Committee of Inquiry into Human Embryology ascribed to the Chief Rabbi which was, in fact, moderate in tone compared with some of the abuse to which members of the Inquiry had been, and are still, subjected both collectively and individually, since the publication of our report in July 1984. None of the members of the Inquiry had any doubt that they were concerned with moral issues. But we were not perhaps all of us certain how such issues ought to be approached, and especially how they should be approached by a body set up by Parliament to make recommendations which might lead to legislation. Many of our critics (including, I believe, the Chief Rabbi) have not really addressed themselves to this problem either: the problem of legislation, and its relation to morality, in such controversial fields. Many of them also embarked on their denunciations without having read the report. In the following pages the report is reproduced in its original form. By way of introduction I append a few observations of a general kind on the nature of moral issues, and the relation between such issues and the law. At the end of the report, I add some notes of a more specific nature about what was expected of this particular Committee of Inquiry, and what may happen as a result of our deliberations.

I do not believe that there is a neat way of marking off moral issues from all others; some people, at some times, may regard things as matters of moral right or wrong, which at another time or in another place are thought to be matters of taste, or indeed to be matters of no importance at all. But it seems likely that in any society, at any time, questions relating to birth and death and to the establishing of families are regarded as morally significant. It was therefore clear from the start that we, the Inquiry, were dealing with moral problems.

The philosopher Hume, in the *Treatise of Human Understanding* (1738) wrote that morality was "more properly felt than judg'd of". He argued that moral distinctions, the basic distinctions between right and wrong, were drawn by moral sense and not by reason. Most ordinary people agree with Hume. Faced with an unfamiliar possibility or a new practice, they reflect on it, and say "I simply feel that it is wrong." Those who discuss moral decisions in terms of what is or is not compatible with the dictates of conscience are, at least in part, appealing to an inner sense of what is or is not tolerable behaviour.

Some people, it is true, are inclined to regard morality not so much as a matter of feeling or sentiment, as of obedience to certain established rules. But even for these people the subjects we were concerned with on the Inquiry presented grave difficulties. For how could rules exist to regulate things like the creation of embryos in the laboratory, which had simply not been envisaged even a decade ago? If morality is indeed obedience to rules, then the rules were yet to be invented.

An alternative and superficially attractive theoretical solution to the problem of how to arrive at moral decisions is offered by utilitarianism. The principle of utility lays down, as the foundation of morality, that an act is right if it benefits more people than it harms, wrong if the balance is the other way. Many scientists engaged in research using human embryos, or doctors employing new techniques to remedy infertility have recourse, wittingly or unwittingly, to utilitarian arguments to justify what they are doing. They point to the immense increase in human happiness when a hitherto infertile couple, like the parents of Louise Brown, manage to have a child; and they argue that there is no pain caused to anyone to weigh in the balance against this happiness. Again, research using embryos may bring unknown benefits in the control of inherited or genetically related disease, and no-one is harmed by such research. Now there are some respects in which a Committee of Inquiry such as ours has to argue on utilitarian presumptions, especially with regard to legislation. I shall discuss this below, but it is necessary to point out first that in a very obvious way the principle of utility cannot solve, by itself, the essential moral problem with regard to research using human embryos on which, in turn, programmes of *in vitro* fertilisation depend. For such research does manifestly harm the embryos. If a strict utilitarian says that embryos do not count, for the purposes of calculation of pleasures and pains, harms and benefits, he is, in saying this, making a moral decision about *how to regard embryos*; and this decision has to be made before any such calculation becomes morally relevant.

By themselves, then, neither utilitarianism nor a blind obedience to rules could solve the moral dilemmas the Inquiry was faced with. We were bound to have recourse to moral sentiment, to try, that is, to sort out what our feelings were, and to justify them. For that a decision is based on sentiment by no means entails that arguments cannot be adduced to support it. Nor are utilitarian arguments based on possible benefits and harms ruled out. It is only that they will not suffice alone. What is essential is to recognise that sentiment has some part, and indeed a crucial part, in arriving at moral decisions. For if this is recognised, it may be less surprising that agreement is not always possible in matters of morality. We know that people's feelings differ. Therefore moral conflict may be unavoidable. If morality were really a question of weighing up harms and benefits, there would be more hope of agreement; and if it were a case of obeying certain rules, we ought to be able to find out what the rules lay down, and come to an agreed decision. In real life morality is more complicated and more various than that. There is no single "correct" view.

If anything, I was more impressed by the extent of moral agreement than of disagreement among members of the Committee of Inquiry, especially considering how many different professions, religions and races we had among our number. But of course we were not set up simply to utter moral pronouncements, agreed or otherwise. We were supposed to advise Ministers with a view to future legislation. Our critics, in Parliament and outside, have frequently forgotten this. We have been accused of making recommendations which attempt a compromise between incompatible moral positions; of proposing arbitrary limits; or of suggesting that things offensive to numbers of people should be legally permissible. But the law is not, and cannot be, an expression of moral feeling. It must apply to everyone, whatever their feelings; it must be both intelligible and enforceable. We were bound, if we were to fulfill our task, to bear in mind the differences between the law and morality. On the other hand, we had, obviously, to recognise their interconnection.

The relation between morality and the law has been a central issue in jurisprudence for very many years. There is a distinction between the way we approached this issue in the two parts of our report, that concerned with the treatment of infertility and that concerned with research. If the question is what measures to remedy infertility should be permitted in this country, the problem may be put in the following form: Why should the law intervene to prevent people using whatever methods are possible to enable them to have children? Why should not everybody be entitled to whatever is currently the best and most efficient treatment for infertility? The issues here are quite closely parallel to the issues raised in the 1960s by the Wolfenden Report on homosexuality between consenting males. Ought the law to intervene to make such conduct criminal or ought it not? The famous view of Lord Devlin (*The Enforcement of Morals*, Oxford, 1959) was that where there is a consensus of opinion against a certain practice among members of the general public (exemplified by the notorious "man on the Clapham omnibus") then the law must intervene to prevent conduct which is repellent to that public. A shared moral view, Lord Devlin argued, was the cement that bound society together. If such shared views were not reflected in law, if law did not enforce what society held to be morally right and wrong, then society itself would disintegrate. A society is characterised by a shared moral view; without it there would be no society. Therefore to act against such a shared view would be tantamount to treason. The law could no more permit acts contrary to the shared morality than it could permit treason.

The drawback with Devlin's view is that, increasingly, we are compelled to accept that "common morality" is a myth. There is no agreed set of principles which everyone, or the majority, or any representative person, believes to be absolutely binding, and especially is this so in areas of moral concern which are radically and genuinely new. We saw that the concept of a "rule" breaks down, in novel and hitherto unthought-of cases, and the notion that there is a consensus morality in such cases is equally untenable. The question must be recast: In situations where people disagree with each other as to the rights and wrongs of a specific form of behaviour, how do we decide whether or not the law is to intervene?

H L A Hart (*Law, Liberty and Morality*, Oxford, 1963) identified two moral problems, on "primary" and the other "critical". At the first level the question is whether a certain practice (homosexual acts between consenting males, or AID) is morally right or wrong; at the second level the question is whether, if the law intervened on this matter, the infringement of liberty involved would itself be morally right or wrong. If we consider a case that concerned the Inquiry, the case of AID, it is plain that moral opinions about it vary through the whole spectrum, from those who think it absolutely wrong (like members of the Jewish Community, who think that it is "bringing orphans into the world", and therefore necessarily wrong) through those who are doubtful, because of the possible risks to AID children, to those who regard it as an absolute right that anyone should have access to AID, whether they are married or single, hetero- or homosexual.

Furthermore, any law enacted to render AID a criminal offence, besides going against the moral views of a fair number of the community, would involve, in itself, a disagreeable intrusiveness, for AID is something that can relatively easily be carried out at home, without any medical intervention. For a law to be enforceable, there would need to be a band of snoopers or people ready to pry into the private lives of others, which might well itself constitute a moral wrong.

Similarly, in the controversial matter of surrogate mothers, the Inquiry agreed unanimously that they disapproved of the practice (largely because of possible consequences for the child); but they also agreed that it could not be prevented by law, because of the intrusiveness of any law that would be enforceable. The Inquiry therefore concentrated on how surrogacy for commercial purposes might be checked, leaving on one side the question whether surrogacy was intrinsically morally right or wrong. We might all of us have answered the primary moral question in a way which made surrogacy wrong. This did not pre-empt the answer to the second-order moral question; Should the law be invoked to stop surrogacy? We all agreed that it would be morally wrong to envisage a law which would intrusively curtail human freedom, and which would in addition be impossible to enforce (how could the law tell whether the child whom Abraham claimed as his own was born to Sara, or to a servant girl who happened to be more fertile?) The Inquiry, then, while unanimously answering the first-order question negatively, holding that surrogacy was wrong, nevertheless held that legislation should not be invoked to prevent it. We did however by a majority recommend that the commercial use of surrogacy arrangements, as a way of making money for an agency, could and should be made a criminal offence. For not only was the wrongness of surrogacy compounded by its being exploited for money, but also a law against agencies would not be intrusive into the private lives of those who were actually engaged in setting up a family.

Thus in some cases it was necessary to distinguish the issue of moral right or wrong, as we saw it, from a further, also moral question, whether it would be right to enforce a moral view, even if such a view were agreed. There was, however, a more testing kind of question, infinitely more important, in my opinion. This was the question of research using human embryos. I have already suggested reasons for the extreme difficulty of reaching an agreement on this matter. Utilitarianism could, as I have argued, by itself provide no solution, simply because the very question at issue was whether or not embryos count as those whose harms and benefits, pleasures and pains, have to be thrown into the balance to be weighed against the benefits or harms to society as a whole. But here we had, it seemed, an issue on which legislation must be foreseen, and must be enacted quickly. No-one felt inclined to argue that the decision whether or not to embark on research with the use of human embryos was a matter of personal conscience, as they might in the case of AID, surrogacy, or, for that matter, homosexuality between adults. Everyone agreed that this was a matter on which there must be legislation, and that whether and to what extent embryos should be used must be a decision for the law.

The reason for this certainty, for the distinction, that is, between what might be thought a private matter and one which was *necessarily* public was somewhat obscure. Nor did the Inquiry draw the distinction explicitly or clearly. But the grounds for it are something like this: research is largely publicly funded. Therefore society, from whom ultimately funding comes, is entitled to know, and even to some extent to control, what research methods are used. If it were revealed after years of work that a number of human embryos had been used to achieve a particular advance in knowledge, the public would still feel that they should have known in advance what research methods were being used; the actual processes and development of the research should have been monitored, and subjected to public scrutiny. This view may be exaggerated; but it is widely held. Society, insofar as it is a single identifiable body, has here, perhaps uniquely, a corporate reaction. It is one of fear. People generally believe that science may be up to no good, and must not be allowed to proceed without scrutiny, both of its objectives and of its methods. There are some things which, manifestly, society would not like to occur in its laboratories. Nor would people be prepared to allow that, even if all such work in laboratories relying on public funds (such as the laboratories of the Medical Research Council) were brought to an end, it could continue in privately funded laboratories. There is a strong feeling that certain possible experiments and research should be subject to criminal law and made a criminal offence, wherever undertaken.

To suggest that it would be all right provided only that it were not publicly financed would be like saying that certain kinds of experiments on patients, let us say children, should be banned from the NHS hospitals but might be permitted in the private sector. I do not believe that the question of individual freedom enters here into public thinking. A scientist who argued that he must be free to carry out whatever research he liked, by whatever methods, would not get much public support, if this involved the use of other human beings. Society feels, albeit obscurely, that its members, especially the most helpless, such as children and the very old, must be protected against possible exploitation by enthusiastic scientists: and embryos are brought into the category of those deserving protection, just as animals are. This is a matter of public, and widely shared, *sentiment*.

Here, then, is an area different from the first. In the case of methods of treating infertility, or of establishing a family, there was a fairly strong view that the freedom of the individual to take what steps he could had to be respected. In addition, as we have seen, the enforcement of a law would in any case be intrusive and would provide, in itself, a hazard to individual liberty. In the case of research, on the other hand, there was general agreement that the issue of individual liberty did not arise. We were confronted here with an area of general moral consensus, with no countervailing arguments against legal enforcement. Perhaps this distinction is not sufficiently brought out in the report itself.

However, as becomes clear from the report and the dissenting opinions appended to it, the degree of protection that the law should afford to the human embryo was not unanimously agreed. Some held that an embryo, being human, should be granted the full protection of the law, and should indeed be treated as though it were no different from a child or an adult. Just as children may not be used in experiments, or for the purposes of research, even if their parents were willingly to permit it, so embryos ought on this view to be totally protected. The majority of the Inquiry held, on the contrary, that its stage of development made an important difference to the degree of protection that should be afforded to a human embryo.

According to the majority view, the question was not, as is often suggested, whether the embryo was alive and human, or whether, if implanted, it might eventually become a full human being. We conceded that all these things were true. We nevertheless argued that, in practical terms, a collection of four or sixteen cells was so different from a full human being, from a new human baby or a fully formed human foetus, that it might quite legitimately be treated differently. Specifically we argued that, unlike a full human being, it might legitimately be used as a means to an end that was good for other humans, both now and in the future.

This, then, was a matter of judgment; and no-one would deny that it was a moral judgment. What was being weighed up was certain human goods on the one hand and the status of these collections of cells on the other. One was to be valued against the other. The majority of the Committee was not moved by the argument that these cells could, if certain conditions were satisfied, become human beings. They did not rely, that is to say, as the minority did, on "potentiality", but on the consideration of what the embryo was at a particular time, its actual mode of existence immediately after fertilisation. If, on broadly utilitarian grounds, the benefits from the use of embryos at this stage seemed very great, and if not only was there no harm in the sense of immediately felt pain to the embryo but also in addition there were no absolute outrage of general moral sentiment (as there would be, for instance, if even a very young or profoundly defective child were used for research) then the majority argued that the embryo might be used for research. The precise point of dispute within the committee was not on the value that should be attached to human life in general, but to the value that should be attached to human life at its very earliest stage of development. It was here that it was necessary to invoke the law. The Committee was not advocating that any embryo, at any stage of its development, should be used as material for research: everyone would have regarded that as morally outrageous. The proposition was that, if the resulting benefits were manifest, an embryo at a particular and very early stage might be used. Therefore there must be a law so drafted as to provide a definition of "very early". We recommended, for reasons set out in the report, a limit of fourteen days. The point was not however the exact number of days chosen, but the absolute necessity for there being a limit set on the use of embryos, in terms of a number of days from fertilisation. In this way the law would be clear. If the limitation on research were set in terms of stage of development or the capacity of the embryo to feel pain, then these limits might be subject to dispute. If the limit is in terms of days, on the other hand, this is a simple matter of counting, and there can be no dispute. This was the reasoning of the Committee.

It was clear then, as I have said, that we had here a genuine moral disagreement, one with regard to fundamental values, within the Committee itself. The law cannot reflect this disagreement. It must come down on one side or the other. But it is important to emphasise that the dispute is not, as has sometimes been suggested, between those who hold that human embryos should never be used for research and those who hold that they may always be used. It is between those who hold that they may never be used, and those who hold that they may be used only subject to stringent regulation and control.

All members of the Committee wanted the criminal law to be invoked in this matter. Members were therefore agreed that there must be a means of enforcing the law, whatever it was, and that this would entail the establishing of an inspectorate, whose task would be to monitor laboratory work in human biology, genetics and embryology. The difference is whether some work involving live embryos should be licensed or none. Those of us who argued for the licensing of some work using human embryos were not, I think, unduly moved by the fact that such work has been going on for a long time up and down the country, nor by the thought that if it were altogether banned from this country many scientists would go abroad to continue it. We tried as far as possible to put such considerations on one side and to consider the matter purely as a question of moral values.

All the other issues we had to consider seemed relatively trivial compared with this one, concerned as it is with a matter which nobody could deny is of central moral significance, the value of human life. Without agreed rules (and it is, as I have already said, idle to pretend that there *are* rules, somehow already laid down, which tell us what to do in these wholly unfamiliar matters) and without any agreed feeling except the feeling that some regulation or other had to be introduced, the Committee was obliged to use a mixture of utilitarian considerations and of judgment. We were obliged moreover to bear in mind that any law must be generally seen to be beneficial, that it must be intelligible and that it must be enforceable. The law must not outrage the feelings of too many people; but it cannot reflect the feelings of them all. It must therefore be drawn with a view to the common good, however this notoriously imprecise goal is to be identified. This was the task that, especially in the second part of the report, the Committee had to tackle. It was a task, as I have suggested, which raised profound and far-reaching questions about the relation between the law and the morality of society.

FOREWORD

1. Our Inquiry was set up to examine, among other things, the ethical implications of new developments in the field. In common usage, the word "ethical" is not absolutely unambiguous. It is often used in the context, for example, of medical or legal ethics, to refer to professionally acceptable practice. We were obliged to interpret the concept of ethics in a less restricted way. We had to direct our attention not only to future practice and possible legislation, but to the principles on which such practices and such legislation would rest.

2. Members of the Inquiry were reluctant to appear to dictate on matters of morals to the public at large. They were also keenly aware that no expression of their own feelings would be a credible basis for recommendations, even if they all felt exactly alike. As our reading of the evidence showed us, feelings among the public at large run very high in these matters; feelings are also very diverse; and moral indignation, or acute uneasiness, may often take the place of argument. But that moral conclusions cannot be separated from moral feelings does not entail that there is no such thing as moral reasoning. Reason and sentiment are not opposed to each other in this field. If, as we believe, it was our task to attempt to discover the public good, in the widest sense, and to make recommendations in the light of that, then we had, in the words of one philosopher, to adopt "a steady and general point of view". So, to this end, we have attempted in what follows to *argue* in favour of those positions which we have adopted, and to give due weight to the counter-arguments, where they exist.

3. Our emphasis on the arguments may make it appear that there was a uniformity of approach and moral feeling in the Inquiry. The reality however has been that our personal feelings and reactions have been as diverse as those presented in the evidence. Some members have a clear perception of the family and its role within society; in considering the various techniques before us their focus has been on the primacy of the interests of the child, and on upholding family values. Other members have felt equally strongly about the rights of the individual within society. Whatever our original feelings and reactions, we have all found that our feelings changed and were modified as work progressed and as we examined the evidence in more

1

detail. This has been a further reason for basing our views on argument rather than sentiment, though we have necessarily been mindful of the truth that matters of ultimate value are not susceptible of proof.

4. A strict utilitarian would suppose that, given certain procedures, it would be possible to calculate their benefits and their costs. Future advantages, therapeutic or scientific, should be weighed against present and future harm. However, even if such a calculation were possible, it could not provide a final or verifiable answer to the question whether it is *right* that such procedures should be carried out. There would still remain the possibility that they were unacceptable, whatever their long-term benefits were supposed to be. Moral questions, such as those with which we have been concerned are, by definition, questions that involve not only a calculation of consequences, but also strong sentiments with regard to the nature of the proposed activities themselves.

5. We were therefore bound to take very seriously the feelings expressed in the evidence. And, as we have said, it would be idle to pretend that there is not a wide diversity in moral feelings, whether these arise from religious, philosophical or humanist beliefs. What is common (and this too we have discovered from the evidence) is that people generally want *some principles or other* to govern the development and use of the new techniques. There must be *some* barriers that are not to be crossed, *some* limits fixed, beyond which people must not be allowed to go. Nor is such a wish for containment a mere whim or fancy. The very existence of morality depends on it. A society which had no inhibiting limits, especially in the areas with which we have been concerned, questions of birth and death, of the setting up of families, and the valuing of human life, would be a society without moral scruples. *And this nobody wants.*

6. In recognising that there should be limits, people are bearing witness to the existence of a moral ideal of society. But in our pluralistic society it is not to be expected that any one set of principles can be enunciated to be completely accepted by everyone. This is not to say that the enunciating of principles is arbitrary, or that there is no shared morality whatever. The law itself, binding on everyone in society, whatever their beliefs,

is the embodiment of a common moral position. It sets out a broad framework for what is morally acceptable within society. Another philosopher put it thus: "The reasons that lead a reflective man to prefer one ... legal system to another must be moral reasons: that is he must find his reasons in some order of priority of interests and activities, in the kind of life that he praises and admires". In recommending legislation, then, we are recommending a kind of society that we can, all of us, praise and admire, even if, in detail, we may individually wish that it were different. Within the broad limits of legislation there is room for different, and perhaps much more stringent, moral rules. What is legally permissible may be thought of as the minimum requirement for a tolerable society. Individuals or communities may voluntarily adopt more exacting standards. It has been our business, however, to recommend how the broad framework should be established, within our particular area of concern.

7. We realise that some people may think that we have set the limits, or have suggested that the barriers be erected, in the wrong places. But at least we hope that we have stated clearly what we think should be done, and exposed, as far as possible, the reasoning that lay behind our recommendations.

8. Barriers, it is generally agreed, must be set up; but there will not be universal agreement about where these barriers should be placed. The question must ultimately be what kind of society can we praise and admire? In what sort of society can we live with our conscience clear?

CHAPTER ONE

THE GENERAL APPROACH

Background to the Inquiry

1.1 The birth of the first child resulting from the technique of *in vitro*[1] fertilisation in July 1978 was a considerable achievement. The technique, long sought, at last successful, opened up new horizons in the alleviation of infertility and in the science of embryology. It was now possible to observe the very earliest stages of human development, and with these discoveries came the hope of remedying defects at this very early stage. However there were also anxieties. There was a sense that events were moving too fast for their implications to be assimilated. Society's views on the new techniques were divided between pride in the technological achievement, pleasure at the new-found means to relieve, at least for some, the unhappiness of infertility, and unease at the apparently uncontrolled advance of science, bringing with it new possibilities for manipulating the early stages of human development.

1.2 Against this background of public excitement and concern, this Inquiry was established in July 1982, with the following terms of reference:

> "To consider recent and potential developments in medicine and science related to human fertilisation and embryology; to consider what policies and safeguards should be applied, including consideration of the social, ethical and legal implications of these developments; and to make recommendations."

Scope of the Inquiry

1.3 In considering our terms of reference, we recognised that we were being asked to examine a sphere of activity still developing, and rapidly changing. A common factor linking all the developments, recent or potential, medical or scientific, was the anxiety which they generated in the public mind. We have therefore looked at the new processes of assisted reproduction,

---

[1] This report distinguishes between *in vitro* meaning "in a glass", and *in vivo* meaning "in the body".

including surrogacy, which can cause public concern. We have also considered artificial insemination, which, though practised in this country for many years, is not universally accepted ethically, nor indeed regulated by law. There were, however, some matters which, though in some sense related, fell outside our terms of reference. Chief among these were abortion and contraception. We have not concerned ourselves directly with these, although the present state of the law in relation to them has been a necessary point of reference in discussions.

1.4 Within the terms of reference we were given two words that had to be clarified. The first of these was *embryology*. While the term "embryo" has been variously defined in considering human embryology, we have taken as our starting point the meeting of egg and sperm at fertilisation. We have regarded the embryonic stage to be the six weeks immediately following fertilisation which usually corresponds with the first eight weeks of gestation counted from the first day of the woman's last menstrual period.

1.5 The second word in need of clarification was *potential*. The pace of scientific discovery is unpredictable. Indeed, a number of major developments has taken place during the lifetime of the Inquiry. The changes which take place in society itself are also difficult to predict. The impact of scientific discoveries on the society of the future is therefore doubly hard to predict. We took the pragmatic view that we could react only to what we knew, and what we could realistically foresee. This meant that we must react to the ways in which people now see childlessness and the process of family formation, taking into account the range of views encompassed by our pluralistic society, the nature and value of clinical and scientific advances and the benefits of research.

Methods of working

1.6 We found it convenient to divide our task into two parts. The first concerned processes designed to benefit the individual within society who faced a particular problem, namely infertility; the second concerned the pursuit of knowledge, much of it designed to benefit society at large rather than the individual. The distinction is not absolute. One cannot divorce pursuit of an individual's goals from the goals of society as a whole and, moreover, policies undertaken for the public good while they may well also benefit individuals can, on the other hand, impose limitations on them. Nonetheless, we found it a useful division, and the report thus deals first with the alleviation of infertility, and second with scientific developments.

1.7 We recognised that within society there is a multiplicity of views on the issues before the Inquiry. We therefore decided to seek evidence from as many organisations, reflecting as many different perspectives, as possible. A list of those who submitted evidence is included as the Appendix. We are particularly grateful for all the time and trouble taken by those who prepared submissions and for the insight they gave us into the problems we were asked to consider. But even with submissions from so many organisations we have to record with regret that we did not receive evidence from as wide a range of minority and special interest groups as we would have liked, despite our best endeavours.

The international dimension

1.8 Anxiety about the implications of the new developments in assisted reproduction is not confined to the United Kingdom. While there is an obvious attraction in a unity of approach to difficult ethical issues, and we have tried as far as possible to keep in touch with developments around the world, there are, in our view, sound reasons for not pursuing this unity of approach at the present time. Different countries are at different stages in the development both of services and of a policy response. They have different cultural, moral and legal traditions, influencing the way in which a problem is tackled and the ways in which it might be resolved. We have therefore made recommendations which we believe to be appropriate specifically in the United Kingdom. Nonetheless, we hope that others may find our proposals of value, just as we have benefitted from the experience of other countries. We accept that there is a case for an international approach. This approach will be best formulated, however, when individual countries have formed their own views, and are ready to pool knowledge and experience.

The role of the Inquiry

1.9 We have confined our recommendations to certain practical proposals, capable of implementation. We have tried to frame these recommendations in general terms, leaving matters of detail to be worked out by Government and other appropriate organisations. We have also indicated what we consider should be matters of good practice. We have clearly indicated where our formal recommendations, if accepted, would require legislative change. The development of science and medical technology in the field of human fertilisation opens up many new issues for the law. *In vitro* fertilisation, for example, has brought about situations not previously contemplated, in relation to which there is either no law at all, or such law as exists was designed for entirely different circumstances. We believe that new laws will be necessary to cope with the new techniques for alleviating infertility and their consequences, and to deal with the developments in research in the field of embryology. But we foresee real dangers in the law intervening too fast and too extensively in areas where there is no clear public consensus. Furthermore both medical science and opinion within society may advance with startling rapidity.

1.10 We do not discuss in the following chapters every situation which might arise and then relate it to all existing law. We have had neither the time nor the resources to do this; nor, in our view, would such a course have been appropriate. Rather we have considered the fundamental questions there raised in relation to any existing law and confined ourselves to what we regard as essential legislative changes. We wish to stress our view that the changes which we propose should apply equally throughout the United Kingdom of Great Britain and Northern Ireland.

CHAPTER TWO

INFERTILITY: THE SCOPE AND ORGANISATION OF SERVICES

2.1 In the past, there was considerable public ignorance of the causes and extent of infertility, as well as ignorance of possible remedies. At one time, if a couple were childless, there was very little they could do about it. Generally the cause of infertility was thought to be something in the woman which made her childless; only occasionally was it thought that there might be something wrong with the man. Even today, there is very little factual information about the prevalence of infertility. A commonly quoted figure is that one couple in ten is childless, but accurate statistics are not available, nor is it known what proportion of this figure relates to couples who choose not to have children. In certain religious and cultural traditions, infertility was, and still is, considered sufficient grounds for divorce. In our own society childless couples used to be advised to adopt a child. Now, as a result of improved contraception, the wider availability of legal abortion and changed attitudes towards the single mother, far fewer babies are placed for adoption.

2.2 Childlessness can be a source of stress even to those who have deliberately chosen it. Family and friends often expect a couple to start a family, and express their expectations, either openly or by implication. The family is a valued institution within our present society: within it the human infant receives nurture and protection during its prolonged period of dependence. It is also the place where social behaviour is learnt and where the child develops its own identity and feeling of self-value. Parents likewise feel their identity in society enhanced and confirmed by their role in the family unit. For those who long for children, the realisation that they are unable to found a family can be shattering. It can disrupt their picture of the whole of their future lives. They may feel that they will be unable to fulfil their own and other people's expectations. They may feel themselves excluded from a whole range of human activity and particularly the activities of their child-rearing contemporaries. In addition to social pressures to have children there is, for many, a powerful urge to perpetuate their genes through a new generation. This desire cannot be assuaged by adoption.

2.3 Arguments have been put to us both for and against the treatment of infertility. First, we have encountered the view that in an over-populated world it is wrong to take active steps to create more human beings who will consume finite resources. However strongly a couple may wish to have children, such a wish is ultimately selfish. It has been said that if they cannot have children without intervention, they should not be helped to do so. Secondly, there is a body of opinion which holds that it is wrong to interfere with nature, or with what is perceived to be the will of God. Thirdly, it has been argued that the desire to have children is no more than a wish; it cannot be said to constitute a need. Other people have genuine needs which must be satisfied if they are to survive. Thus services designed to meet these needs must have priority for scarce resources.

2.4 In answer to the first point, it is never easy to counter an argument based on the situation of the world as a whole with an argument relying on the desires of individuals. We saw it as our function to concentrate on individuals rather than on the world at large. Questions about the distribution of resources within the world as a whole lie far outside our terms of reference. In any event, the number of children born as a result of techniques to assist in the treatment of infertility will always be insignificant in comparison with the naturally increasing world population. On the second point, the argument that to offer treatment to the infertile is contrary to nature fails to convince in view of the ambiguity of the concepts "natural" and "unnatural". We took the view that actions taken with the intention of overcoming infertility can, as a rule, be regarded as acceptable substitutes for natural fertilisation. Thirdly, the argument that the desire to have children is only a wish, not a need, and therefore should not be satisfied at the expense of other more urgent demands on resources can be answered in several ways. There are many other treatments not designed to satisfy absolute needs (in the sense that the patient would die without them) which are readily available within the NHS. Medicine is no longer exclusively concerned with the preservation of life, but with remedying the malfunctions of the human body. On this analysis, an inability to have children is a malfunction and should be considered in exactly the same way as any other. Furthermore infertility may be the result of some disorder which in itself needs treatment for the benefit of the patient's health. Infertility is not something mysterious, nor a cause of shame, nor necessarily something that has to be endured without attempted cure. In addition, the psychological distress that may be caused by infertility in those who want children may precipitate a mental disorder warranting treatment. It is, in our view, better to treat the primary cause of such distress than to alleviate the symptoms. In summary, we conclude that infertility is a condition meriting treatment.

Eligibility for treatment

2.5 It is sometimes suggested that infertility treatment should be available only to married couples, in the interests of any child that may be born as a result. While we are vitally aware of the need to protect these interests, we are not prepared to recommend that access to treatment should be based exclusively on the legal status of marriage.

2.6 In discussing treatment for infertility, this report takes the term *couple* to mean a heterosexual couple living together in a stable relationship, whether married or not. We use the words *husband* and *wife* to denote a relationship, not a legal status (except where the context makes differentiation necessary, for example in relation to legitimacy).

2.7 In the evidence, concern was expressed that infertility treatment may be provided for couples without due regard for the interests of any child that may be born as a result. For example the couple may have a previous conviction for child abuse. It has been argued that the greater the degree of intervention in the creation of a child, the more responsibility must be taken for that child. However the evidence also drew attention to the absence of any restrictions on procreation by fertile couples, whatever their circumstances. Indeed, some of the evidence referred to the fact that Articles 8 and 12 of the European Convention on Human Rights guarantee a respect for family life and the right to found a family. It has been argued that these provisions create a right to take full advantage of the techniques which are available to alleviate infertility.

2.8 There are other considerations which many believe should be taken into account. For example, a woman may seek treatment when she has herself, at an earlier stage, been sterilised at her own request. Perhaps because of a new marriage, she now very much wants children. The question may be raised whether, if she has children, albeit from another marriage, she should be eligible for infertility treatment. Again, a woman who has had a child may subsequently become infertile. Opinions may be divided about whether she should be eligible for treatment.

2.9 Furthermore, the various techniques for assisted reproduction offer not only a remedy for infertility, but also offer the fertile single woman or lesbian couple the chance of parenthood without the direct involvement of a male partner. To judge from the evidence, many believe that the interests of the child dictate that it should be born into a home where there is a loving, stable, heterosexual relationship and that, therefore, the *deliberate* creation of a child for a woman who is not a partner in such a relationship is morally wrong. On the other side some expressed the view that a single woman or lesbian couple have a right under the European Convention to have children even though those children may have no legal father. It is further argued that it is already accepted that a single person, whether man or woman, can in certain circumstances provide a suitable environment for a child, since the existence of single adoptive parents is specifically provided for in the Children Act 1975.[1]

2.10 In the same way that a single woman may believe she has a right to motherhood, so a single man may feel he has a right to fatherhood. Though the feminist position is perhaps more frequently publicised, we were told of a group of single, mainly homosexual, men who were campaigning for the right to bring up a child. Their primary aim at present is to obtain in practice equal rights in the adoption field, but they are also well aware of the potential of surrogacy for providing a single man with a child that is genetically his. There have been cases in other countries of surrogacy in such circumstances. It can be argued that as a matter of sex equality if single women are not totally barred from parenthood, then neither should single men be so barred.

2.11 We have considered these arguments, but, nevertheless, we believe that as a general rule it is better for children to be born into a two-parent family, with both father and mother,

---

[1] Section 11 of the Children Act 1975

although we recognise that it is impossible to predict with any certainty how lasting such a relationship will be.

2.12 We have considered very carefully whether there are circumstances where it is inappropriate for treatment which is solely for the alleviation of infertility to be provided. In general we hold that everyone should be entitled to seek expert advice and appropriate investigation. This will usually involve referral to a consultant. However, at the present time services for the treatment of infertility are in short supply, both for initial referral and investigation and for the more specialised treatments considered in this report. In this situation of scarcity some individuals will have a more compelling case for treatment than others. In the circumstances medical practitioners will, clearly, use their clinical judgment as to the priority of the individual case bearing in mind such considerations as the patient's age, the duration of infertility and the likelihood that treatment will be successful. So far this is not contentious. However, notwithstanding our view that every patient is entitled to advice and investigation of his or her infertility, we can foresee occasions where the consultant may, after discussion with professional health and social work colleagues, consider that there are valid reasons why infertility treatment would not be in the best interests of the patient, the child that may be born following treatment, or the patient's immediate family.

2.13 This question of eligibility for treatment is a very difficult one, and we believe that hard and fast rules are not applicable to its solution. We recognise that this will place a heavy burden of responsibility on the individual consultant who must make social judgments that go beyond the purely medical, in the types of case we have discussed. We considered whether it was possible for us to set out the wider social criteria that consultants, together with their professional colleagues, should use in deciding whether infertility treatment should be provided for a particular patient. We decided it was not possible to draw up comprehensive criteria that would be sensitive to the circumstances of every case. We recognise however that individual practitioners are on occasions going to decline to treat a particular patient and **we recommend that in cases where consultants decline to provide treatment they should always give the patient a full explanation of the reasons.** This would at least ensure that patients were not kept in ignorance of the reason for refusal, and would be able to exercise their right to seek a second opinion.

Organisation of services

2.14 We recognise the difficulty of providing reliable statistics on infertility because of the number of infertile couples who do not seek treatment or are voluntarily childless. Nevertheless we were surprised at how few data there were on the prevalence of infertility, the extent of available services, their location and the numbers treated. Where figures were available, they were often out of date and of dubious relevance. Quite often, people with an infertility problem seek professional advice about other symptoms. Thus any estimate of the extent of infertility treatment within the NHS understates the present level of provision; the primary diagnosis may reflect the symptoms about which advice was first sought, rather than infertility. We believe that these data deficiencies should be remedied so that policy makers and planners can make decisions against a background of objectively assessed facts. **We recommend that funding should be made available for the collection of adequate statistics on infertility and infertility services.**

2.15 The infertile, and those representing their interests, indicated in evidence to the Inquiry considerable dissatisfaction with the present pattern of services. Patients tend to feel that, unless they attend one of the limited number of specialist infertility clinics, their problem is somehow tangential to the mainstream activity in the gynaecological clinic; they feel that not'enough attention is paid to the stressful nature of their condition; they complain about a lack of continuity of care, a lack of any sense of urgency in determining the cause of their problem, a tendency to see the woman and the man separately rather than together as a couple and a shortage of services for investigation and treatment of infertility in men.

2.16 We find the present haphazard organisation of services unsatisfactory. While we can appreciate that all gynaecologists want to offer help to their own patients, we nonetheless believe that a greater degree of specialisation is necessary. A working party of the Royal College of Obstetricians and Gynaecologists (RCOG) has recommended[1] the creation of a new sub-specialty of reproductive medicine which would include infertility, and though we regard an assessment of the merits of this proposal as outside our terms of reference, we see some advantages in it. **We recommend that each health authority should**

---

[1] Report of the RCOG Working Party on Further Specialisation within Obstetrics and Gynaecology November 1982.

review its facilities for the investigation and treatment of infertility and consider the establishment, separate from routine gynaecology, of a specialist infertility clinic with close working relationships with specialist units, including genetic counselling services, at regional and supraregional level. Where it is not possible to have a separate clinic we recommend that infertility patients should be seen separately from other types of gynaecological patient wherever possible. The husband and wife should be seen together and it would then be possible for the necessary expertise to be available to deal with problems in the man as well as the woman. It would allow numbers of infertile couples to meet each other, and would offer scope for developing informal arrangements for mutual support. A more specialised service would, we believe, make the best use of available expertise and resources.

Relative priorities

2.17 While the determination of relative priorities is not a matter for this Inquiry, we note with concern the lengthy hospital waiting lists for gynaecological treatment and the tendency in some places for infertility patients to be given the lowest priority on waiting lists for both in-patient and out-patient treatment. A reorganisation designed to promote a more effective delivery of services need not necessarily involve, in the long term, much greater expenditure. We recognise, however, that in some authorities, where little has been provided till now, a certain amount of new expenditure on infertility services will be entailed. In order to facilitate local planning, **we recommend the establishment of a working group at national level made up of central health departments, health authorities and those working in infertility, to draw up detailed guidance on the organisation of services.**

2.18 We urge that the priorities argument should not be used to cover up the present lack of systematic planning for infertility services. We recognise that the needs and resources of individual health authorities will vary, but **recommend that consideration be given to the inclusion of plans for infertility services as part of the next round of health authority strategic plans.**

14

CHAPTER THREE

TECHNIQUES FOR THE ALLEVIATION OF INFERTILITY: COMMON THREADS

3.1 In the following chapters we shall be discussing remedies for infertility. Apart from questions raised about the ethics of these methods, and their implications for those who propose to use them, there are several common threads running through them all, of which we consider three below. As a preliminary we would stress that treatment for infertility should be undertaken under the supervision of a registered medical practitioner.

Anonymity

3.2 A number of the techniques we consider involves a third party outside the infertile couple. In artificial insemination by donor (AID) another man provides the semen; in egg donation another woman provides the egg; in embryo donation both another man and another woman contribute; in surrogacy another woman provides her uterus (womb) for the duration of the pregnancy. In all cases, the question is whether it is better that a third party who helps a couple to overcome their infertility should be known to the couple or that the third party should remain anonymous. On rare occasions a brother or a sister may be the most appropriate person to give help, but our general view is that anonymity protects all parties not only from legal complications but also from emotional difficulties. **We recommend that as a matter of good practice any third party donating gametes[1] for infertility treatment should be unknown to the couple before, during and after the treatment, and equally the third party should not know the identity of the couple being helped.**

Counselling

3.3 A second issue concerns the counselling, advice, information and discussion that should be available for those who seek treatment for infertility. Many of the problems which may arise in the course of treatment, whether this treatment ends in the birth of a child or not, are complex and they need to be given careful consideration over a period of time. We therefore believe

---

[1] Gamete is the collective term used to describe both sperm and eggs.

that counselling should be available for infertile couples and for donors. In particular the task of the doctor and the counsellor must be to ensure that couples and donors fully understand the implications of what they are embarking on, what rights and duties they may have, and where they may expect to experience difficulties.

3.4 The counselling that we envisage is essentially non-directional. It is aimed at helping individuals to understand their situation and to make their own decisions about what steps should be taken next. Counselling need not necessarily take place at the hospital, though this may be the most convenient location. It should be carried out in a neutral atmosphere and involve a skilled, fully trained counsellor. **We recommend that counselling should be available to all infertile couples and third parties at any stage of the treatment, both as an integral part of National Health Service provision and in the private sector.** We recognise that there may not be sufficient counsellors trained in this field at present, but we feel it is possible for counsellors trained in other fields to adapt their skills to deal with infertility. Specialised further training and funding for those attending such courses will need to be made available. We look to training bodies in social work and counselling to give guidance on these training needs and how they should be met.

Consent

3.5 We feel it to be very important that time and consideration should be devoted to explaining fully to prospective patients and, where necessary, to their partners the details of any infertility treatment they are to undergo. No such treatment should be undertaken without the fully informed consent of the patient and this should, in the case of more specialised treatment, normally be obtained in the presence of someone not associated with the performance of the procedures. **We recommend that in the case of more specialised forms of infertility treatment the consent in writing of both partners should be obtained, wherever possible, before treatment is begun, as a matter of good practice. Any written consent should be obtained on an appropriate consent form.** It also seems desirable that the process of explaining and describing prospective treatment should be embarked upon as far in advance as possible so that both partners have plenty of time to discuss and consider the treatment.

CHAPTER FOUR

TECHNIQUES FOR THE ALLEVIATION OF INFERTILITY *cont'd*:

I Artificial insemination

4.1 The term artificial insemination (AI) is used to refer to the placing of semen inside a woman's vagina or uterus by means other than sexual intercourse. The principle of this technique has been known for centuries in the veterinary context. The simplicity of artificial insemination contrasts sharply with the technical complexity of more recent developments such as *in vitro* fertilisation. It begins with the collection of semen from the husband or a donor, through masturbation. The semen is either placed in the upper part of the vagina next to the cervix or injected into the uterus through a fine catheter. Insemination is undertaken near the predicted time of ovulation, the time in a woman's menstrual cycle when she has the highest chance of conceiving. The semen used may be fresh or it may have been previously frozen and thawed before use.

Artificial insemination by husband (AIH)

4.2 This technique is used for some couples who cannot otherwise conceive, but where the man is not completely infertile. For example, it may be felt that the chances of pregnancy would be increased by concentrating the husband's semen or by inserting it directly into the uterus. When the husband is severely physically disabled and unable to achieve intercourse, AIH may offer the only possibility for him to father a child. It may further be used when the husband cannot ejaculate during intercourse. AIH may also be used to overcome a particular type of female infertility known as cervical hostility where the sperm are killed or rendered inactive by the cervical mucus. In such cases AIH may be successful if the semen is injected into the uterus. There are also situations where a man may have his semen frozen and stored for later use in artificial insemination, because he is to undergo surgery or treatment such as chemotherapy or radiotherapy that may result in sterility or damage to the testes.

Arguments against AIH

4.3 Opposition to AIH is founded on the view that it represents an unwarranted deviation from natural processes of intercourse. Those who hold this view argue also that the unitive and procreative aspects of sexual intercourse should not be separated. And it is argued that it involves the practice of masturbation which is held to be wrong. We acknowledge the sincerity with which these views are held, although we ourselves do not share them. People who hold them will clearly not wish to seek AIH for themselves.

The Inquiry's view

4.4 The majority of views expressed to us however, saw AIH as an acceptable form of treatment, where clinically indicated. We ourselves see no moral objection to its practice. We believe that where there is the intention to bring about the birth of a child and this takes place within the context of a stable relationship, such intervention is acceptable. It is simply a means of bringing together the sperm and egg of a husband and wife so that fertilisation can take place *in vivo*. Nevertheless we have grave misgivings about AIH in one type of situation. A man who has placed semen in a semen bank may die and his widow may then seek to be inseminated (see Chapter Ten). This may give rise to profound psychological problems for the child and the mother.

4.5 We see little need for, or practical possibility of, formal regulation of AIH. However we hold that AIH, like other treatments for infertility, should be administered by, or under the supervision of, a medical practitioner registered under the Medical Act, 1983. The use of fresh semen for AIH, can, in our opinion, be regulated by a professional code of practice. Where frozen semen is used, the procedures which we recommend in Chapter Ten should apply.

Artificial insemination by donor (AID)

4.6 Artificial insemination by donor (AID) may be used when investigations have shown the husband to be sterile or to have significantly reduced fertility, or it may be used for the avoidance of hereditary diseases when these are carried by the male (9.2 and 9.3). In this procedure the woman is inseminated with semen from a donor.

Attitudes to AID

4.7 The first formal public comment on AID in this country came with the publication of the Archbishop of Canterbury's report[1] on artificial insemination in 1948. The Archbishop himself was highly critical of the practice of AID, though not of AIH, recommending that it should be made a criminal offence. However no action was taken in this direction. In 1960 the Feversham Committee, set up by the Government to consider AI, reported;[2] it considered that AIH was an acceptable form of treatment for some couples, but believed that the majority within both society and the medical profession was opposed to the practice of AID. It concluded that AID was an undesirable practice, strongly to be discouraged. Since 1960 the practice of AID has continued to grow. In 1968, the then Minister for Health decided that AIH and AID should be available within the NHS if recommended on medical grounds. The increase in requests for information about AID and where it was provided led the British Medical Association to set up a panel in 1971 under the chairmanship of Sir John Peel to look into the medical aspects of human artificial insemination. This panel reported in 1973[3] and recommended that, for the small proportion of couples for whom AID would be appropriate, the practice should be available within the NHS at accredited centres. No action was taken to establish a system of accreditation.

4.8 In the decade since the Peel panel reported the trend of increasing acceptability and demand for AID has continued. In 1982, the latest year for which figures are available, the Royal College of Obstetricians and Gynaecologists knew of over 1000 pregancies conceived and at least 780 live births following AID in this country. This is undoubtedly an under-estimate. But we were not able to find detailed information about AID services. NHS centres are not required to identify themselves in any of the returns that health authorities make to the Health Departments, though there are several centres where AID is provided under NHS auspices which are well-established and

---

[1] Artificial Human Insemination: the report of a Commission appointed by His Grace the Archbishop of Canterbury. Society for the Propagation of Christian Knowledge, 1948.

[2] Home Office and Scottish Home Department. Departmental Committee on Human Artificial Insemination. Report. (Chairman: The Earl of Feversham). HMSO, 1960 (Cmnd 1105).

[3] British Medical Association. Annual Report of the Council. Appendix V: Report of the Panel on Human Artificial Insemination. (Chairman: Sir John Peel). British Medical Journal Supplement, 1973, 7 April, vol. II, p 3–5.

whose existence is widely known. In addition there is a number of private centres, particularly in London, providing AID and the British Pregnancy Advisory Service offers AID at some of its pregnancy advice bureaux, located throughout the country.

The present position

4.9 Under existing law neither AIH nor AID is unlawful. A child born to a married couple as a result of AIH is the legitimate child of that couple. A child born as a result of AID, on the other hand, is illegitimate, and so is liable to suffer all the disadvantages associated with that status. In theory the husband of the woman who bears an AID child has no parental rights and duties in law with regard to that child; these in principle lie with the donor, who could be made liable to pay maintenance, and who could apply to a court for access or custody.

Arguments against AID

4.10 Submissions to the Inquiry included some expressing strongly-held views against the practice of AID. There are objections derived from the view that AID represents the introduction of a third party into what ought to be an exclusive relationship. This is held to be morally wrong in itself, whatever the motives of those involved may be. But it is also seen as a threat to the relationship and to the family which is based on it. The threat arises because the child would be biologically the wife's and the donor's, and the husband would have played no physical part in its procreation. Some go so far as to suggest that the introduction of a third party into the marriage means that AID is in fact comparable to adultery, in that it violates the exclusive physical union of man and wife, and represents a break in the marriage vows. However, in law AID does not constitute adultery[1] and in practice there are several distinctions. AID involves no personal relationship between the mother and the donor at all, and the identity of the true father of the AID child will normally be unknown to the mother, and unascertainable by her. In most cases it can be assumed that the mother's husband is willing from the start to treat any resulting child as his own and not merely as an accepted

---

[1] MacLennan v MacLennan 1958 S.C 105.

"child of the family". It will often be true that AID with the consent of the husband is a mark of stability in a marriage while an act of adultery may well be the opposite.

4.11 The question remains as to whether in AID the introduction of a third party nevertheless constitutes a threat to the marriage. It is argued that the wife may feel that the child was hers rather than her husband's and that her husband had in some sense failed her. Similarly, the husband may experience a sense of inadequacy and of exclusion because he has not participated in the creation of the child. In consequence the wife may be emotionally closer than the husband to the child, and this may threaten the couple's relationship. There are, however, existing parallels, for example, that of a step-parent, where relationships in which one parent is not genetically related to the child can work extremely well. We do not accept that the donor is *necessarily* a threat to the stability of the relationship.

4.12 We have examined the position of the child in AID, and particularly the possible dangers to the child which some people regard as so threatening that they oppose the use of AID altogether. Certainly, if a child is desired *simply* to preserve a marriage, the outlook for that child may be poor. Moreover AID has tended, partly because of the legal situation, to be surrounded with secrecy. This secrecy amounts to more than a desire for confidentiality and privacy, for the couple may deceive their family and friends, and often the child as well. Indeed couples who achieve pregnancy may come to look on their AID child as a true child of the marriage. However the sense that a secret exists may undermine the whole network of family relationships. AID children may feel obscurely that they are being deceived by their parents, that they are in some way different from their peers, and that the men whom they regard as their fathers are not their real fathers. We have little evidence on which to judge this. But it would seem probable that the impact on children of learning by accident that they were born as a result of AID would be harmful—just as it would be if they learned by accident that they were adopted or illegitimate. However, while we agree that it is wrong to deceive children about their origins, we regard this as an argument against current attitudes, not against AID in itself.

4.13 Furthermore there is anxiety about the frequency with which semen from an individual donor is used. One fear is that a donor may pass on to future generations any inherited condition from which he suffers or of which he is a carrier. This can be avoided by proper screening procedures designed to ensure that men with dominant[1] conditions are identified and excluded from being donors. The risk of passing on a recessive[2] condition depends on the number of children a donor fathers. Another fear consistently expressed is that AID children may unwittingly enter into an incestuous relationship or contract a marriage within the prohibited degrees, though the true medical and genetic consequences of inadvertent incest or marriage within the prohibited degrees are often over-stated. The risks from all these problems can be largely reduced by limiting the number of children fathered by one donor.

4.14 Those who are anxious about the consequences of AID for the individuals who are involved also express concern about the implications for society at large and in particular for the family. It is not possible to predict future consequences of the growth in the practice of AID but we would point out that those engaging in AID are, in their own view, involved in a positive affirmation of the value of the family.

Arguments for AID

4.15 Many of the arguments against AID can be countered, as we have shown. In addition to these counter arguments, however, there are several points directly in favour of AID. AID enables couples to have a child whom they can bring up as their own and who is biologically the wife's. It is not a particularly invasive process. It is essentially simple and painless: no anaesthesia or surgery is required. It is an out-patient treatment requiring only regular visits to the clinic. If a woman continues AID treatment for a period of time, the success rate is similar to that of natural insemination, and this may be very important for a couple already in their thirties or suffering acutely from the distress of childlessness. An AID child is a child very much wanted: a couple may have had to endure years of waiting and will consequently cherish the child. The fact that the couple share the experience of pregnancy, in the

---

[1] A "dominant" condition is one in which the disorder will manifest itself in all individuals who possess the gene responsible for the condition.

[2] A "recessive" condition will manifest itself only in an individual who has received the gene from both parents. In the case of an individual inheriting a recessive gene from only one parent that individual will not normally manifest any of the symptoms of the disorder, but will be a carrier of that recessive gene.

same way as any other couple does, may strengthen their relationships as joint parents. Many of the submissions made to the Inquiry were strongly in favour of AID.

.

The Inquiry's view

4.16 We have concluded that AID should no longer be left in a legal vacuum but should be subject to certain conditions and safeguards, and receive the protection of the law. It is certain that, for some people, AID will always remain unacceptable. Nevertheless we cannot accept their objections as a reason for denying the opportunity for treatment to those infertile couples who do not share their beliefs. Moreover the practice of AID will continue to grow, with or without official sanction and its clandestine practice could be very harmful. It is therefore desirable that AID should be available as a treatment for the alleviation of infertility, in a form subject to all possible safeguards. We regard it as a legitimate form of treatment for those infertile couples for whom it might be appropriate. Therefore **we recommend that AID should be available on a properly organised basis and subject to the licensing arrangements described in Chapter Thirteen, to those infertile couples for whom it might be appropriate. Consequently we recommend that the provision of AID services without a licence for the purpose should be an offence.**

Principles of AID provision and consequential legal changes

4.17 There is a number of principles which we suggest must underlie the practice of AID. The English Law Commission recommended that the law should be reformed to remove all the legal disadvantages of illegitimacy so far as they affect the illegitimate child. Thus there would be no legal distinction between legitimate and illegitimate children. Both parents would have equal rights unless and until a court ordered otherwise. The Commission further recommended that when a married woman had received AID treatment with her husband's consent, the husband, rather than the donor should, for all legal purposes, be regarded as the father of a child conceived by AID. We unanimously agree and accordingly **recommend that the AID child should in law be treated** as the legitimate child of its mother and her husband where they have both consented to the treatment. This will require legislation.

4.18 We consider that every donor must be screened to exclude, as far as possible, hereditary diseases and infections that could be passed either to the child or to the mother (such as sexually transmitted diseases or hepatitis B), and to identify the donor's rhesus factor. A full medical examination of the donor should also be undertaken.

4.19 It is the practice of some clinics in the USA to provide detailed descriptions of donors, and to permit couples to exercise choice as to the donor they would prefer. In the evidence there was some support for the use of such descriptions. It is argued that they would provide information and reassurance for the parents and, at a later date, for the child. They might also be of benefit to the donor, as an indication that he is valued for his own sake. A detailed description also offers some choice to the woman who is to have the child, and lack of such choice can be said to diminish the importance of the woman's right to choose the father of her child.

4.20 The contrary view, also expressed in the evidence, is that detailed donor profiles would introduce the donor as a person in his own right. It is also argued that the use of profiles devalues the child who may seem to be wanted only if certain specifications are met, and this may become a source of disappointment to the parents if their expectations are unfulfilled.

4.21 As a matter of principle we do not wish to encourage the possibility of prospective parents seeking donors with specific characteristics by the use of whose semen they hope to give birth to a particular type of child. We do not therefore want detailed descriptions of donors to be used as a basis for choice, but we believe that the couple should be given sufficient relevant information for their reassurance. This should include some basic facts about the donor, such as his ethnic group and his genetic health. A small minority of the Inquiry, while supporting the principle set out above, and without compromising the principle of anonymity, consider that a gradual move towards making more detailed descriptions of the donor available to prospective parents, if requested, could be beneficial to the practice of AID, provided this was accompanied by appropriate counselling. **We recommend that on reaching the age of eighteen the child should have access to the**

basic information about the donor's ethnic origin and genetic health and that legislation be enacted to provide the right of access to this. This legislation should not be retrospective.

4.22 We were agreed that there is a need to maintain the absolute anonymity of the donor, though we recognise that in privately arranged donation, for example between brothers, a different situation would of course apply; such domestic arrangements, however, fall outside any general regulation. Anonymity would give legal protection to the donor but it would also have the effect of minimising the invasion of the third party into the family. Without anonymity, men would, it is argued, be less likely to become donors in view of the risk that they might subsequently be identified and forced to accept parental responsibility for an AID child, by payment of maintenance or otherwise. Clearly in view of our recommendation (4.17) that the AID child should for all purposes be treated as the legitimate child of the couple who have benefitted from successful treatment, the donor should have no responsibilities towards the child. **We therefore recommend a change in the law so that the semen donor will have no parental rights or duties in relation to the child.** We recognise that one consequence of this provision would be that AID children, even if informed about the circumstances of their conception would never be entitled to know the identity of their genetic fathers.

4.23 Another principle on which AID should be based is that of joint consent, that is, a joint decision by the man and woman to seek the treatment. We believe strongly that both must consent to the woman being inseminated with the semen of another man. In giving consent, care must be taken that both the woman and the man fully understand and agree that the selection and screening of the donors will be undertaken by the medical practitioner. **We recommend that the formal consent in writing by both partners should, as a matter of good practice, always be obtained before AID treatment begins. A consent form should be used and thoroughly explained to both partners.**

4.24 In the case of married couples we considered whether the law needed to impose requirements as to the form in which the husband's consent should be given. **We recommend, following the English Law Commission, that it should be presumed that the husband has consented to AID,**

unless the contrary is proved. The legal status of the AID child should not have to depend on proof of consent to treatment or on the existence of a document evidencing consent. In other words, the burden of proof should rest on the husband to show he has not consented. However, we appreciate that where it is shown that the husband has not consented, the effect of our recommendation (see 4.22) that the donor should have no parental rights and duties in relation to the AID child will mean that in the eyes of the law the child will have no father. We regard this as inescapable, and the same situation will arise where AID is provided to an unmarried woman. The law will be recognising what in many cases is already the *de facto* situation.

4.25 As matters stand at present there is a temptation for the couple to conceal the true situation when a child is conceived as a result of AID, in order to hide the fact that the husband is infertile and to avoid unfavourable reactions among relatives and friends. Therefore the couple may, in registering the birth, state that the husband is the father, thus committing an offence.[1] Where the mother is married and the husband consents to AID (4.17) **we recommend that the law should be changed so as to permit the husband to be registered as the father.** We are fully aware that this can be criticised as legislating for a fiction since the husband of a woman who has conceived by AID will not be the genetic father of the child and the register of births has always been envisaged as a true genetic record. Nevertheless it would in our view be consistent with the husband's assuming all parental rights and duties with regard to the child. However we are of the view that consideration should be given as a matter of urgency to making it possible for the parents in registering the birth to add "by donation" after the man's name.

4.26 There are several other practical points to be considered in relation to AID. One is the question of limiting the number of children that an individual may father because of the remote possibility of unwitting incest between children of the same donor, and because of risks of transmission of inherited disease, (4.13). We decided that there was no conclusive argument for any particular figure, and we also recognised the practical difficulties of ascertaining numbers of live births, especially when

---

[1] Section 4 of the Perjury Act 1911 (England and Wales) Section 53 of the Registration of Births, Deaths and Marriages (Scotland) Act 1965.

frozen semen is used. However we were agreed that some limit should be imposed, and we favour a limit of ten children, although we consider this a factor that the licensing body should keep under regular review. **We recommend for the present a limit of ten children who can be fathered by donations from any one donor.** To prevent the possibility of the same donor being used unwittingly by different clinics, **we recommend that the NHS numbers of all donors be checked by the clinics where they make their donations against a new centrally maintained list of NHS numbers of existing donors, which is to be held separately from the NHS central register.** In this way the anonymity of the donor could be preserved but the number of children he had fathered could be recorded. The basic information about the donor which would be made available to the child at the age of eighteen would also be held on the central record of AID donors.

4.27 We have heard from many sources about the difficulty of finding semen donors. It is our hope that this problem will diminish with growing public acceptance of AID, and with the legal changes we have recommended. We were however interested to hear of the way in which the French AID system recruits new donors. Prospective recipients of AID are asked to approach married couples among their friends with a view to persuading them to make a donation, not for the use of any particular recipient, to the semen bank. This approach seems to us to have several benefits: it spreads the appeal for donors to a broader section of the community; it emphasises the donation aspect, and couples rather than individuals are party to the donation. We heard of a strong dependence in some UK clinics on students for donations and we are concerned that a young man may in later years find the fact that he has made donations difficult to discuss with his wife and children. An argument has also been put to us that the only way to attract sufficient donors in this country is to offer a fee. The practice of the payment of donors varies considerably at the moment. It is something about which we are uneasy, given the atmosphere in which AID is practised. We are concerned that the offer of a fee may tempt some men to withhold from the doctor details that would, if known, make them unacceptable as donors. Further we feel that the offering of a fee could encourage some men to offer their semen to a number of different clinics though this practice should be prevented by our proposals in 4.26. **We recommend that there should be a gradual move towards a system where semen donors should be given only their expenses.**

4.28 We believe that people should be encouraged to be open about this form of treatment. Such openness may be easier in consequence both of the legal changes we have recommended, and of the increase in provision which we hope to see. Together these should make AID more acceptable as a means of relieving male infertility. But a change in attitude towards male infertility is also required.

CHAPTER FIVE

TECHNIQUES FOR THE ALLEVIATION OF INFERTILITY *cont'd:*

II In Vitro Fertilisation

5.1 Unlike AID, *in vitro* fertilisation (IVF) is very much a new development. Of those women who are infertile a small proportion can produce healthy eggs but, although they have a normal uterus, have damaged or diseased fallopian tubes which prevent the egg passing from the ovary to the uterus. A certain proportion of these women can be helped by tubal surgery. Until IVF became a reality, the possibility of achieving a pregnancy for women with tubal problems was not great. IVF may be appropriate perhaps for 5% of infertile couples. Recently claims have been made for IVF as a treatment for other forms of infertility including its use in the treatment of oligospermia[1] and unexplained infertility.

5.2 The concept of IVF is simple. A ripe human egg is extracted from the ovary, shortly before it would have been released naturally. Next, the egg is mixed with the semen of the husband or partner, so that fertilisation can occur. The fertilised egg, once it has started to divide, is then transferred back to the mother's uterus. In practice the technique for recovery of the eggs, their culture outside the mother's body, and the transfer of the developing embryo to the uterus has to be carried out under very carefully controlled conditions. The development of laparoscopic[2] techniques during the 1960s made the collection of the egg, in cases where the ovaries were accessible, relatively easy. (Another technique for egg recovery based on ultrasound identification[3] has now been developed.) It was

---

[1] Oligospermia is the term used to describe semen in which the number of sperm present is reduced or markedly reduced compared with the number of sperm present in normal semen.

[2] The laparoscope is an optical surgical instrument which is used to inspect the internal abdominal and pelvic organs so that minor surgical procedures can be performed including the recovery of one or more eggs from those ovarian follicles that are ripe. Laparoscopy usually requires a general anaesthetic but does not usually involve an overnight stay in hospital.

[3] Ultrasound can now be used to identify the position of a ripe follicle containing an egg. A needle is then passed through the woman's abdominal wall and other organs and is guided to the follicle by use of ultrasound. The egg is then withdrawn through the needle. This technique can be used under local anaesthetic and can be used to recover more than one egg at a time.

not particularly difficult to fertilise the human egg *in vitro*. The real difficulty related to the implantation of the embryo in the uterus after transfer. A pregnancy achieved in this way must not only survive the normal hazards of implantation of *in vivo* conception, but also the additional problems of IVF and embryo transfer. More is now known about how best to replicate the natural sequence of events, but undoubtedly achieving a successful implantation is still the most uncertain part of the procedure.

5.3 Because of these difficulties it is common practice to transfer more than one embryo to the potential mother whenever possible, and for this reason several eggs need to be recovered. This is achieved by artificial stimulation, known as superovulation, of the woman's ovaries to ensure that she produces several eggs in one cycle. After an appropriate course of drugs, as many ripe eggs as are accessible are harvested just before the time of ovulation. Each egg is then mixed with semen to achieve fertilisation. Assuming there is no abnormality in the semen, the success rate of fertilisation is usually at least 75%. Some embryos may however show signs of poor or abnormal development; when the time comes to transfer the embryos to the woman it may be that there is only one embryo suitable for transfer, or there may be several.

5.4 The case for transferring more than one embryo is that this should give the woman a better chance of achieving a pregnancy. There is also an argument that if two or more embryos are transferred each helps the other towards implantation. However, if too many embryos are transferred and they all implant this may result in a multiple pregnancy with all the added risks of such a pregnancy including the risks of miscarriage, premature delivery and resulting immaturity at birth. There are differences of opinion about how many embryos should be transferred, given these risks. This is a field where constant reassessment is needed as new evidence becomes available. We have considered arguments that a limit should be imposed on the total number of embyos that should be transferred on each occasion, but we believe that in each individual case the number of embryos to be transferred must be a matter of clinical judgment on the part of the practitioner responsible for the woman's care. This responsibility should be made clear in the consent form. In addition to the technical arguments we have outlined, a practitioner must also give very serious consideration to the social problems for the family that may follow the birth of more than twins, problems that may affect the continuing health and wellbeing of the mother in looking after the children and may adversely affect the children themselves.

5.5 Despite the technical difficulties of IVF, at the time we write, there have been some hundreds of such births throughout the world. These births continue to exercise considerable fascination. At the same time, this public interest creates, in itself, difficulties, adding to the pressure on doctors practising in this field who are not only trying to provide a new treatment for their patients, but are also constantly working in the public eye.

Arguments against IVF and responses

5.6 Although many people regard IVF as an exciting new possibility for helping the childless, there are those who are deeply worried by its development. This opposition can be categorised as opposition either based on fundamental principles, or based on the consequences of the practice of IVF. The fundamental arguments against IVF are the same as those against AIH—that this practice represents a deviation from normal intercourse and that the unitive and procreative aspects of sexual intercourse should not be separated. Those who hold this view believe that this is an absolute moral principle which must be upheld without exception. This view is sincerely and strongly held. As a question of individual conscience, there will be those who will not wish to receive this form of treatment nor participate in its practice, but we would not rely on those arguments for the formulation of a public policy.

5.7 The arguments against IVF based on a consideration of the consequences are more varied; but those who put forward such arguments may take as their starting point the acceptance of IVF as a legitimate form of treatment for infertility. Their reservations start when IVF results in more embryos being brought into existence than will be transferred to the mother's uterus. They argue that it is not acceptable deliberately to produce embryos which have potential for human life when that potential will never be realised. As we have noted above the opinion of the medical profession on the whole is that in the present state of knowledge superovulation is very desirable. But if more embryos are brought into existence than are transferred, it is held to be morally unacceptable to allow them to die.

5.8 Another argument against IVF is that which draws an analogy between IVF and heart transplants, or other forms of "high technology" medical care, and asks whether the country can afford such expensive treatment which benefits only a few, and whether money could not be "better" spent, that is, with beneficial effects for more people, elsewhere. While we accept that questions about the uses of resources are proper questions, deserving serious consideration, essentially they relate to the extent of provision, not to whether there should be any provision at all. Further, without some provision of a service there can be no opportunity to evaluate the real costs and benefits of a technique, nor can the technique be refined and developed so as to become more cost-effective. The priorities argument is, in our view, an argument for controlled development, not an argument against the technique itself.

Arguments for IVF

5.9 The positive argument in favour of IVF is simple: the technique will increase the chances for some infertile couples to have a child. For some couples this will be the only method by which they may have a child that is genetically entirely theirs.

The Inquiry's view

5.10 We have reached the conclusion that IVF is an acceptable means of treating infertility and **we therefore recommend that the service of IVF should continue to be available subject to the same type of licensing and inspection as we have recommended with regard to the regulation of AID** (see Chapter Four). For the protection and reassurance of the public this recommendation must apply equally to IVF within the NHS and in the private medical sector. At the present time IVF is available on a limited scale within the NHS and **we recommend that IVF should continue to be available within the NHS.** One member of the Inquiry would not like to see any expansion of NHS IVF services until the results obtained in using this technique are more satisfactory. IVF requires a concentration of skilled medical and scientific expertise, and it is appropriate for only a small proportion of infertile couples. Therefore we would not argue that it should be available at all district general hospitals, or even at all university teaching hospitals. However in order to minimise travelling and other inconvenience to patients, we believe that ultimately

NHS centres should be distributed throughout the UK. We recognise that there will be those who will press for at least one in every region.

5.11 We are conscious that such specialised units with their distinctive organisational features, would have considerable cost implications, and we are mindful of the priorities argument mentioned above. We are also mindful that IVF is only one of a range of treatments for infertility and, as suggested in Chapter Two there is scope for improvement in the provision of infertility services generally. We would not want to see IVF, with its present relatively low success rate, cream off all the resources available for the treatment of infertility just because it has the glamour of novelty. Details of the financing of the service are outside our terms of reference, but these factors make it desirable that the early development of the service within the NHS be carefully monitored. **We recommend that one of the first tasks of the working group, whose establishment we recommend in 2.17 should be to consider how best an IVF service can be organised within the NHS.** There will be continuing development of private IVF clinics alongside those within the NHS, but we believe it is important that there should be a sufficient level of NHS provision for childless couples not to feel that their only recourse is to the private sector.

5.12 In order to put IVF into perspective we are particularly concerned that an accurate estimate of success is given, because childless couples develop high expectations of the technique. We do not want the unhappiness and disappointment they may have already experienced to be exacerbated by false or unrealistic hopes. It is now very difficult to give an estimate of the success of the technique because of differing methods of measuring success and also because rates vary between centres. However we have been given permission by Mr Steptoe and Dr Edwards to quote the following figures on the outcome of IVF treatment carried out at Bourn Hall Clinic, as an illustration. During the period October 1980 (when the clinic opened) to the end of December 1983, 2,388 laparoscopies were carried out for 1,234 women of whom 690 were admitted for treatment on two or more occasions. These resulted in a total of 362 pregnancies, of which 105 ended in miscarriage and four in an ectopic pregnancy. Of these 362 pregnancies, in 271 treatment was undertaken because of diseased or absent fallopian tubes without associated semen problems. The majority of the remainder were undertaken either because of a combination of semen problems and diseased fallopian tubes or because of semen problems alone.

5.13 In 1983 there were 967 laparoscopies performed for 579 women. In 934 of these laparoscopies one or more eggs was recovered, and in 762 one or more eggs was fertilised. In all these cases one or more embryos was transferred to the woman and in 192 a pregnancy occurred which ended in birth or a clinically recognisable miscarriage.[1]

5.14 By May 1984 the clinic knew of 439 pregnancies, of which 131 were ongoing. 215 children had been born since it had opened, including 18 sets of twins and one set of triplets. Among these infants there had been no major congenital malformations.

5.15 It seems to us that the technique has now passed the research stage and can be regarded as an established form of treatment for infertility.

---

[1] This total does not include "biochemical pregnancies" where early tests following embryo transfer suggest that implantation might have occurred, but there is no subsequent clinical evidence of pregnancy.

CHAPTER SIX

TECHNIQUES FOR THE ALLEVIATION OF INFERTILITY *cont'd*:

III Egg Donation

6.1 Egg donation has been attempted in the United States of America and in Australia, where there has been one live birth. This procedure may help those women who cannot themselves produce an egg. It may also help those who would be candidates for IVF except that in their case egg collection is impossible because their ovaries are inaccessible. About 5% of infertile couples might benefit from the technique. A mature egg is recovered from a fertile woman donor, for example during sterilisation, and is fertilised *in vitro*, using the semen of the husband of the infertile woman. The resulting embryo is then transferred to the patient's uterus. If it implants she may then carry the pregnancy to term. There are other situations where eggs might be donated. When a woman is herself undergoing infertility treatment and several eggs have been recovered from her, she may be prepared to donate one or more eggs to another woman whose infertility can be treated only by egg donation.

6.2 A major feature of the technique is timing. It is essential to monitor closely the donor's menstrual cycle so that egg recovery takes place at the correct time, shortly before the ripe egg would have been released naturally from the ovary. This means that for donors who are giving an egg while undergoing some other treatment, the main operation has to take place at the time dictated by the decision to collect the egg. Such monitoring is complicated and time-consuming, and at present would necessitate the donor attending hospital more frequently than the main operation itself would require. Experience with IVF has shown that reliance on the natural cycle to produce eggs results in a lower success rate than when superovulation is used to stimulate egg production. For egg donation to have much chance of success it would similarly be necessary to induce superovulation in the donor.

6.3 At the present time human eggs cannot be successfully used after freezing and thawing, which means they must be used soon after collection. And so it is necessary not only to time egg collection at the right point in the donor's cycle, but also to have a suitable recipient immediately ready to receive the fertilised egg. The practical problems thus presented limit the applicability of the technique. The problems would be substantially reduced if it became possible to store eggs by freezing (see Chapter Ten). Just as the use of frozen semen in AID permits a greater flexibility, the same would be true for egg donation. The freezing, storing and thawing of eggs is likely to become feasible within a few years. In the future it may be possible to mature eggs *in vitro* that have been recovered at an immature stage.

Arguments against egg donation

6.4 Egg donation is open to the same kinds of objection as AID. There is the same objection to the introduction of a third party into the marriage. There is also concern about the possible impact on the child and the possible harmful effects on society in general. In addition, egg donation involves a considerable degree of intervention in the normal process of fertilisation. In this respect it is similar to IVF. We have examined these views elsewhere. Moreover egg donation can be opposed on grounds of the physical risks involved for the donor, for there is some risk, as there is in any invasive procedure, to the egg donor from the actual removal of eggs.

Arguments for egg donation

6.5 For some couples egg donation provides the only chance of their having a child which the woman can carry to term, and which is the genetic child of her husband. The couple, it is argued, experience the pregnancy as other couples do, and for this reason egg donation has an advantage over AID, in that both partners contribute to the birth of the child.

The Inquiry's view

6.6 In weighing up the arguments for and against egg donation we have concluded that since we have accepted AID and IVF it would be illogical not to accept egg donation, notwithstanding the relatively minor surgical risks to the donor inherent in egg recovery. We consider that egg donation is ethically acceptable where the donor has been properly counselled and is fully aware of the risks. It is both logical and consistent that the law should treat egg donation in the same way as AID and that the same principles of practice described in Chapter Four should apply to both. However, there is an important practical difference between the two procedures. Egg donation requires an invasive procedure to obtain the egg and the whole process necessitates the active assistance of the medical profession. Nonetheless so far as possible similar principles should apply in relation to the anonymity of the donor, screening, donor profiles, the child's right to know the facts of the donation and access for the couples to information about the donor's ethnic origin and genetic health and, similarly, access for the child to this information on reaching the age of majority. **We recommend that egg donation be accepted as a recognised technique in the treatment of infertility subject to the same type of licensing and controls as we have recommended for the regulation of AID and IVF. The principles of good practice we have already considered in relation to these other techniques should apply, including the anonymity of the donor, limitation of the number of children born from the eggs of any one donor to ten, openness with the child about his genetic origins, the availability of counselling for all parties and informed consent.**

6.7 Despite our desire to maintain the anonymity of the donor we recognise that because of the present practicalities of egg donation, particularly the fact that eggs cannot be successfully stored, it may not always at present be possible to achieve this. An exception to the principle of anonymity would occur where the egg was donated by a sister or close friend. In such cases particularly careful counselling for all concerned would be necessary and thought would have to be given as to how and at what stage the child should be told about its parentage.

6.8 Egg donation produces for the first time circumstances in which the genetic mother (the woman who donates the egg), is a different person from the woman who gives birth to the child, the carrying mother. The law has never, till now, had to face this problem. There are inevitably going to be instances where the stark issue arises of who is the mother. In order to achieve some certainty in this situation it is our view that where a woman donates an egg for transfer to another the donation should be treated as absolute and that, like a male donor she should have no rights or duties with regard to any resulting child. **We recommend that legislation should provide**

that when a child is born to a woman following donation of another's egg the woman giving birth should, for all purposes, be regarded in law as the mother of that child, and that the egg donor should have no rights or obligations in respect of the child. We also consider that as with AID (4.25), if the parents so wish, the mother's name may be followed in the birth register by the words "by donation".

CHAPTER SEVEN

TECHNIQUES FOR THE ALLEVIATION OF INFERTILITY *cont'd* :

IV Embryo Donation

7.1 Embryo donation would help the same groups of women who might benefit from egg donation and, more particularly, the even smaller number whose husbands are also infertile. Embryo donation may take two forms. One involves the donation of both egg and semen. The donated egg is fertilised *in vitro* with donated semen and the resulting embryo transferred to a woman who is unable to produce an egg herself and whose husband is infertile. The second method, known as lavage, does not involve removing the egg by surgical intervention. Instead the egg is released naturally from the ovary at the normal time in the donor's menstrual cycle. At the predicted time of ovulation she is artificially inseminated with semen from the husband of the infertile woman (or from a donor if the husband is also infertile). Some three to four days later, before the start of implantation, the donor's uterus is "washed out" and any embryo retrieved is then transferred to the uterus of the infertile woman. If the embryo implants successfully the recipient carries the pregnancy to term. Embryo donation by lavage is, according to its advocates, much safer for the donor as it does not require general anaesthesia, and a simple and safer procedure is involved; moreover, for the embryo, there is the advantage of a shorter interval *in vitro* during which time it might deteriorate. When semen from the husband is used, the child is genetically his though not his wife's.

Arguments against embryo donation

7.2 The objections that are raised in relation to egg donation and AID can also be made to embryo donation, that is, the introduction of a third party into an exclusive relationship, and the possible impact on the child and on society in general. Again, where a surgical procedure is used to recover the egg there is some risk to the donor. Further, where lavage is used, there is a risk of pregnancy in the donor, since the embryo may not be washed out; and of the introduction of infection to the uterus or other problems. A further objection to embryo donation where a semen donor is used is that neither of the nurturing parents has contributed genetically to the child.

Arguments for embryo donation

7.3 In the evidence it was suggested that embryo donation constituted a form of pre-natal adoption, with the advantage over normal adoption that the couple share the experience of pregnancy and childbirth, and, it is further argued, the mother and child experience bonding during pregnancy.

The Inquiry's view

7.4 Embryo donation is probably the least satisfactory form of donation. There is however likely to be a very limited number of cases where a donated egg is fertilised by donated semen *in vitro* and the resultant embryo transferred to the uterus of a woman who would otherwise be unable to have a child. **We therefore recommend that the form of embryo donation involving donated semen and egg which are brought together *in vitro* be accepted as a treatment for infertility, subject to the same type of licensing and controls as we have recommended with regard to the regulation of AID, IVF and egg donation.**

7.5 We do however have some reservations about the use of lavage because of the risk to the egg donor. **We recommend that the technique of embryo donation by lavage should not be used at the present time.**

7.6 It is entirely consistent with our view that donation should lead to negation of all rights and duties that such an embryo once transferred should be regarded for all purposes as that of the carrying mother. Should the risks of donation by lavage be overcome and that technique become acceptable any embryo donated in this way should likewise be treated as that of the woman who carries the pregnancy. **We recommend that the legislation proposed in 4.25 and 6.8 should cover children born following embryo donation.** These recommendations mean that a child born following embryo donation to a married couple will, in the eyes of the law, have that couple as parents. In a case where the carrying mother is unmarried she will, in any event, in the eyes of the law be regarded as the mother of the child. The changes in the law we have earlier proposed would make it possible for the child to be registered, without making a false declaration, in the name of the nurturing parents, thus ensuring the child's legitimacy, assuming they had given informed consent. We also suggest that their names could be followed by the words "by donation" in the birth register, if the parents so wish.

7.7 As with donation and AID there is a number of principles which should underlie the provision of embryo donation—the anonymity of the donor; openness about the treatment, especially with the child; the provision of a full explanation of what is involved to those taking part, including donors, screening and donor profiles, and access for the parents and the child (on reaching the age of majority) to information about the donor's genetic health. These have been fully described in Chapter Four.

CHAPTER EIGHT

TECHNIQUES FOR THE ALLEVIATION OF INFERTILITY *cont'd*:

What is surrogacy?

8.1 Surrogacy is the practice whereby one woman carries a child for another with the intention that the child should be handed over after birth. The use of artificial insemination and the recent development of *in vitro* fertilisation have eliminated the necessity for sexual intercourse in order to establish a surrogate pregnancy. Surrogacy can take a number of forms. The commissioning mother may be the genetic mother, in that she provides the egg, or she may make no contribution to the establishment of the pregnancy. The genetic father may be the husband of the commissioning mother, or of the carrying mother; or he may be an anonymous donor. There are thus many possible combinations of persons who are relevant to the child's conception, birth and early environment. Of these various forms perhaps the most likely are surrogacy involving artificial insemination, where the carrying mother is the genetic mother inseminated with semen from the male partner of the commissioning couple, and surrogacy using *in vitro* fertilisation where both egg and semen come from the commissioning couple, and the resultant embryo is transferred to and implants in the carrying mother.

8.2 There are certain circumstances in which surrogacy would be an option for the alleviation of infertility. Examples are where a woman has a severe pelvic disease which cannot be remedied surgically, or has no uterus. The practice might also be used to help those women who have suffered repeated miscarriages. There are also perhaps circumstances where the genetic mother, although not infertile, could benefit from the pregnancy being carried by another woman. An example is where the genetic mother is fit to care for a child after it is born, but suffers from a condition making pregnancy medically undesirable.

8.3 If surrogacy takes place it generally involves some payment to the carrying mother. Payment may vary between reimbursement of expenses, and a substantial fee. There may, however, be some instances where no money is involved, for example, where one sister carries the pregnancy for another.

The present position

8.4 There is at present no provision for a surrogacy service within the NHS. Private agencies exist in certain other countries and in the UK one agency is said to have started to operate. The practice is not in itself unlawful. None of the parties to a surrogacy arrangement, including any agency operating on a commercial basis, contravenes existing criminal law, unless the terms of the agreement contravene the provisions of adoption law, which prohibit payments in connection with adoption.[1]

8.5 Any surrogacy arrangement would necessarily involve some form of agreement between the parties concerned, however informal. Although it may be assumed that in the majority of cases the agreement would be kept and the matter never brought before a court, it is likely that grave difficulties of enforcement would ensue in the event of a dispute over such an agreement. There is little doubt that the Courts would treat most, if not all, surrogacy agreements as contrary to public policy and therefore unenforceable. Where one party broke the agreement the other party could not expect to invoke the court's assistance. Thus, if the carrying mother changed her mind and decided she wished to keep the child it is most unlikely that a court would order her, because she had previously agreed to do so, to hand over the child against her will. Nor in such a case would a court order the surrogate mother to repay any fee paid to her under the terms of the agreement.

8.6 The Courts do, however, have jurisdiction over children which is quite separate from and independent of the law of contract. Where a court has to consider the future of a child born following a surrogacy agreement, it must do so in accordance with the child's best interests in all the circumstances of the case, and not according to the terms of any agreement between the various adults. The child's interests being the first and paramount consideration, it seems likely that only in very exceptional circumstances would a court direct a surrogate mother to hand over the child to the commissioning couple. The present state of the law makes any surrogacy agreement a risky undertaking for those involved.

---

[1] Section 50 of the Adoption Act 1958.

8.7 Many unforeseen events may occur between the moment of entering into the surrogacy agreement and the time for handing over the child, and these may alter the whole picture. Apart from the most obvious one of the surrogate mother changing her mind, it may, for example, be discovered that the child is handicapped or the commissioning mother may die or become disabled.

8.8 Embryo transfer makes possible for the first time a situation where the carrying mother is not the genetic mother. Where there has been a donation of egg or embryo to the carrying mother we have recommended that the woman who gives birth should, for all purposes in law, be regarded as the mother. The position following surrogacy is far less straightforward. It is not difficult to envisage circumstances where serious arguments could develop as to whether the genetic mother or the carrying mother ought in truth to be regarded as the mother of the child. The resolution of this issue could be of great importance in questions such as inheritance, citizenship or a claim for wrongful death.

The father's position

8.9 We have also considered the case of the commissioning father. In most cases the genetic father will be the husband of the commissioning mother. As regards enforcing any surrogacy agreement to which he is party, the commissioning father faces the difficulties described in 8.5. He may also be vulnerable to a claim by the carrying mother for an affiliation order if she keeps the child and the court might or might not make such an order according to the facts of the particular case. Unless he is married to the carrying mother he will, in the eyes of the law, be treated as an "unmarried" father with all the consequences that ordinarily flow from that.

Arguments against surrogacy

8.10 There are strongly held objections to the concept of surrogacy, and it seems from the evidence submitted to us that the weight of public opinion is against the practice. The objections turn essentially on the view that to introduce a third party into the process of procreation which should be confined to the loving partnership between two people, is an attack on the value of the marital relationship (see 4.10). Further, the intrusion is worse than in the case of AID, since the contribution of the carrying mother is greater, more intimate and personal, than the contribution of a semen donor. It is also argued that it is inconsistent with human dignity that a woman should use her uterus for financial profit and treat it as an incubator for someone else's child. The objection is not diminished, indeed it is strengthened, where the woman entered an agreement to conceive a child, with the sole purpose of handing the child over to the commissioning couple after birth.

8.11 Again. it is argued that the relationship between mother and child is itself distorted by surrogacy. For in such an arrangement a woman deliberately allows herself to become pregnant with the intention of giving up the child to which she will give birth, and this is the wrong way to approach pregnancy. It is also potentially damaging to the child, whose bonds with the carrying mother, regardless of genetic connections, are held to be strong, and whose welfare must be considered to be of paramount importance. Further it is felt that a surrogacy agreement is degrading to the child who is to be the outcome of it, since, for all practical purposes, the child will have been bought for money.

8.12 It is also argued that since there are some risks attached to pregnancy, no woman ought to be asked to undertake pregnancy for another, in order to earn money. Nor, it is argued should a woman be forced by legal sanctions to part with a child, to which she has recently given birth, against her will.

Arguments for surrogacy

8.13 If infertility is a condition which should, where possible, be remedied, it is argued that surrogacy must not be ruled out, since it offers to some couples their only chance of having a child genetically related to one or both of them. In particular, it may well be the only way that the husband of an infertile woman can have a child. Moreover, the bearing of a child for another can be seen, not as an undertaking that trivialises or commercialises pregnancy, but, on the contrary, as a deliberate and thoughtful act of generosity on the part of one woman to another. If there are risks attached to pregnancy, then the generosity is all the greater.

8.14 There is no reason, it is argued, to suppose that carrying mothers will enter into agreements lightly, and they have a perfect right to enter into such agreements if they so wish, just as they have a right to use their own bodies in other ways, according to their own decision. Where agreements are genuinely voluntary, there can be no question of exploitation, nor does the fact that surrogates will be paid for their pregnancy of itself entail exploitation of either party to the agreement.

8.15 As for intrusion into the marriage relationship, it is argued that those who feel strongly about this need not seek such treatment, but they should not seek to prevent others from having access to it.

8.16 On the question of bonding, it is argued that as very little is actually known about the extent to which bonding occurs when the child is *in utero*, no great claims should be made in this respect. In any case the breaking of such bonds, even if less than ideal, is not held to be an overriding argument against placing a child for adoption, where the mother wants this.

The Inquiry's view

8.17 The question of surrogacy presented us with some of the most difficult problems we encountered. The evidence submitted to us contained a range of strongly held views and this was reflected in our own views. The moral and social objections to surrogacy have weighed heavily with us. In the first place we are all agreed that surrogacy for convenience alone, that is, where a woman is physically capable of bearing a child but does not wish to undergo pregnancy, is totally ethically unacceptable. Even in compelling medical circumstances the danger of exploitation of one human being by another appears to the majority of us far to outweigh the potential benefits, in almost every case. That people should treat others as a means to their own ends, however desirable the consequences, must always be liable to moral objection. Such treatment of one person by another becomes positively exploitative when financial interests are involved. It is therefore with the commercial exploitation of surrogacy that we have been primarily, but by no means exclusively, concerned.

8.18 We have considered whether the criminal law should have any part to play in the control of surrogacy and have concluded that it should. We recognise that there is a serious risk of commercial exploitation of surrogacy and that this would be difficult to prevent without the assistance of the criminal law.[1] We have considered whether a limited, non-profit making surrogacy service, subject to licensing and inspection, could

---

[1] See expression of dissent from Dr Greengross and Dr Davies.

have any useful part to play but the majority agreed that the existence of such a service would in itself encourage the growth of surrogacy. **We recommend that legislation be introduced to render criminal the creation or the operation in the United Kingdom of agencies whose purposes include the recruitment of women for surrogate pregnancy or making arrangements for individuals or couples who wish to utilise the services of a carrying mother; such legislation should be wide enough to include both profit and non-profit making organisations. We further recommend that the legislation be sufficiently wide to render criminally liable the actions of professionals and others who knowingly assist in the establishment of a surrogate pregnancy.**

8.19 We do not envisage that this legislation would render private persons entering into surrogacy arrangements liable to criminal prosection, as we are anxious to avoid children being born to mothers subject to the taint of criminality. We nonetheless recognise that there will continue to be privately arranged surrogacy agreements. While we consider that most, if not all, surrogacy arrangements would be legally unenforceable in any of their terms, we feel that the position should be put beyond any possible doubt in law. **We recommend that it be provided by statute that all surrogacy agreements are illegal contracts and therefore unenforceable in the courts.**

8.20 We are conscious that surrogacy like egg and embryo donation may raise the question as to whether the genetic or the carrying mother is the true mother. Our recommendations in 6.8 and 7.6 cover cases where eggs or embryos have been donated. There remains however the possible case where the egg or embryo has not been donated but has been provided by the commissioning mother or parents with the intention that they should bring up the resultant child. If our recommendation in 8.18 is accepted, such cases are unlikely to occur because of the probability that the practitioner administering the treatment would be committing an offence. However, for the avoidance of doubt, we consider that the legislation proposed in 6.8 and 7.6 should be sufficiently widely drawn to cover any such case. If experience shows that this gives rise to an injustice for children who live with their genetic mother rather than the mother who bore them then in our view the remedy is to make the adoption laws more flexible so as to enable the genetic mother to adopt.

CHAPTER NINE

THE WIDER USE OF THESE TECHNIQUES

9.1 So far in this report we have been concerned with the alleviation of infertility. The processes we have considered can, however, also be seen as a facility, a service available to anyone, whether infertile or otherwise, to enable them to have a child in a particular way.

The transmission of hereditary disease

9.2 The increased understanding of genetics and the availability of genetic counselling has meant that people are now aware of the principles that govern the inheritance of genetic diseases and the likelihood of transmitting an hereditary disease which may be severely handicapping in its effects to the next generation, either because the individual has the condition or is a carrier. Couples who know of the possibility of such disorders in either or both families face a difficult choice. For some conditions, prenatal diagnostic screening already provides a means of detecting abnormalities or genetic disorders in the foetus. This may provide parents with an opportunity for termination of pregnancy if they want it. However there are people for whom a termination is unacceptable. For them, the choice at the moment is a harsh one, between the risk of having handicapped children, and having no children at all.

9.3 For such people, the use of a technique involving donated eggs or semen which do not contain the genetic material associated with the hereditary disease offers real hope of giving birth to healthy children. Even though they do not require the donation as a treatment for infertility, it seems to us right that, in their circumstances, they should be offered, as part of the process of genetic counselling, the facility to use a technique which will help to prevent handicap in the next generation. We know that, where the hereditary condition may be transmitted by the male, AID is already quite often suggested. We hope that our proposals for the regulation of AID, and for making the child legitimate, will in the future make this a more acceptable option. We hope, too, that those involved in counselling couples at risk of transmitting an hereditary disease will now begin to consider the potential benefits of egg and, in rare circumstances, embryo donation to overcome problems where the woman is at risk of passing on the hereditary condition. We believe that the range of options for helping such couples should be made more widely known, so that the fears and unhappiness caused through the risk of transmitting an hereditary condition can be eased. **We recommend that it should be accepted practice to offer donated gametes and embryos to those at risk of transmitting hereditary disorders.**

Sex selection

9.4 "Sex selection" is a term which covers two different concepts. It may be used to refer to the choice of the gender of an embryo before fertilisation occurs, or to the identification of the gender of an already existing embryo. Either could be of benefit in avoiding certain sex-linked genetic disorders. Knowledge of foetal sex can be crucial where either member of a couple is known to be the carrier of a sex-linked hereditary disorder such as haemophilia or Duchenne muscular dystrophy. The sex of any child to which they may give birth will determine whether or not the child may have inherited the disorder.

Gender identification

9.5 At present the only techniques for discovering the gender of a foetus before birth which are well established are through the use of high resolution ultra-sound scan, or through the incidental information that can be obtained in carrying out amniocentesis,[1] a diagnostic procedure developed with the aim of screening for neural tube defects and for chromosomal abnormality. Neither procedure can be used before sixteen to eighteen weeks gestation.

9.6 A limited amount of post-implantation gender identification is already taking place when there is the risk of transmitting a sex-linked hereditary disease through the use of amniocentesis; the usual practice is that the possibility of a termination is discussed with the couple if the foetus is of the sex that would be at risk. Amniocentesis has two main disadvantages. Because the procedure cannot be undertaken before sixteen weeks gestation, and the necessary tests may then take

---

[1] This is a procedure in which some of the fluid surrounding the foetus is withdrawn through a fine needle passed into the uterus through the lower abdominal wall.

between ten days and three weeks to complete, if the couple request termination it involves a late abortion with the possible attendant psychological and physical trauma for the mother. There is also a small risk, approximately 1%, that amniocentesis will itself result in miscarriage.

9.7 If it is successfully developed it may be possible to use the technique of chorion biopsy as a means of post-implantation gender identification much earlier in pregnancy, from six to twelve weeks gestation. This new technique involves the removal, usually through the cervix, of a very small part of the foetal membranes (the tissues which surround the embryo in the uterus). After removal, the chorion biopsy can be examined to identify the chromosomes, and hence the gender of the foetus. The potential of chorion biopsy is being evaluated at the present time. The risk of disturbing a pregnancy as a result of the technique is not known, but preliminary studies suggest that some couples might prefer to accept the possible risk in order to be sure that a child will not be born with a sex-linked handicapping condition.

Post-fertilisation and pre-implantation gender identification

9.8 This sort of technique would be applicable only for embryos fertilised *in vitro*. If it is shown that, as in some animal species, one cell can be removed from a human embryo at a very early stage of development without detriment to the embryo's subsequent normal development, it would make gender identification before transfer to the mother's uterus possible. This would probably involve the freezing of the embryo while the isolated cell was examined. In this case, if the sex was that desired, the embryo could be unfrozen and transferred to the mother's uterus in a subsequent cycle. It might in the future become possible to identify the gender of the embryo from a single cell without the need to freeze the embryo until the woman's next menstrual cycle. Pre-implantation gender identification would not involve the mother in any abortion procedure, because embryos of the sex associated with the handicapping condition would not be transferred to her uterus.

Possible future methods of sex selection

9.9 At the time of writing, a considerable amount of research is proceeding to find ways to ensure the conception of a child of a particular sex; none of this research has yet produced a successful method.

9.10 The possibility of separating male- and female-bearing sperm was first suggested many years ago, primarily in the veterinary context. If an effective technique became available that would separate the male- from the female-bearing sperm it would then be possible to use sperm of the chosen type for fertilisation either *in vivo* or *in vitro*. This could be used to prevent the birth of a child with a sex-linked hereditary disease. Despite considerable research and various claims in the medical literature during the past decade that, for example, alteration of the acidity of the secretions in the vagina might vary the likelihood of a male or female child being conceived, none of the methods proposed has yet been shown to be successful.

Other reasons for sex selection

9.11 So far we have discussed the use of sex selection in a clinical context, where it would be practised solely for the purpose of avoiding hereditary sex-linked disorders. We see no reason why, if a method of selecting the sex of a child before fertilisation is developed, this should not be offered to couples who have good medical reasons for choosing the sex of their child. But if an efficient and easy method of ensuring the conception of a child of a particular sex became available, it is likely that some couples would wish to make use of it for purely social reasons. Such a practice would obviously affect the individual family and the children involved, and would also have implications for society as a whole. It is impossible to predict, either in the long or the short term, the likely effects of such a practice on the ratio of males to females within society. It is often suggested that a majority of couples would choose that their first child was male, and if this happened, it could have important social implications, since there is considerable evidence that the firstborn sibling may enjoy certain advantages over younger siblings. It would have particular implications for the role of women in society, although some would argue that these effects would today be less damaging than they might have been a hundred years ago. These important considerations make the Inquiry dubious about the use of sex selection techniques on a wide scale, but because of the difficulty of predicting the outcome of any such trend we have not found it possible to make any positive recommendations on this issue. Nevertheless, we consider that the whole question of the acceptability of sex selection should be kept under review. (See Chapter Thirteen.)

9.12 It seems possible that as a result of the present research in this field, in the not too distant future, a reliable and simple method of selecting the sex of a child before fertilisation will be developed. The apparatus for carrying out such a procedure could well be marketed commercially for self-administration. This seems to us to be an important area of concern. As we understand the current position, there is a possibility that certain types of "do-it-yourself" materials for gender selection would not come within the ambit of the Medicines Act 1968. We consider it essential that the public should be protected from any such kits that do not actually possess the qualities claimed for them and therefore **recommend that all types of "do-it-yourself" sex selection kits should be brought within the ambit of control provided by the Medicines Act with the aim of ensuring that such products are safe, efficacious and of an acceptable standard for use.**

CHAPTER TEN

THE FREEZING AND STORAGE OF HUMAN SEMEN, EGGS AND EMBRYOS

10.1 The freezing, storage and thawing of human semen and embryos for subsequent use in artificial insemination or IVF are already practical realities, but a safe and reliable method of freezing and thawing human eggs has not yet been developed, although this is probably not far in the future. First, we see no objection in principle to the use of freezing in the treatment of infertility. There are however practical problems which may cause concern. There is anxiety that the process of freezing could induce damage in the gametes or embryos in a way which might lead to the birth of a child with an abnormality of structure or function. Nevertheless the experience of using frozen human semen for artificial insemination is reassuring, and so are animal studies in which semen has been used for AI after long-term frozen storage. **We therefore recommend that the use of frozen semen in artificial insemination should continue.**

10.2 This situation is not however paralleled in the case of eggs which have been fertilised after frozen storage. At present human eggs fertilised after freezing and thawing do not develop successfully. In addition, if this difficulty were overcome the problem of whether the resulting embryo would develop normally would still remain to be resolved. So far there is insufficient evidence on which to base a judgement that the freezing and thawing of human eggs will not result in abnormalities. **We therefore recommend that the use of frozen eggs in therapeutic procedures should not be undertaken until research has shown that no unacceptable risk is involved. This will be a matter for review by the licensing body.** (See Chapter Thirteen)

10.3 At the time of writing a small number of pregnancies has been achieved after frozen storage of human embryos, of which at least one has led to a live birth. Animal studies suggest that any damage caused by freezing is more likely to kill the embryo entirely than to impair its development and it is not thought likely that freezing of human embryos will cause abnormalities. Nevertheless, as a matter of good clinical practice, checks should be made after thawing, to ensure so far as possible, that any frozen human embryo which is to be transferred to a woman is developing normally. **We recommend that the clinical use of frozen embryos may continue to be developed under review by the licensing body.** (See Chapter Thirteen)

10.4 The other problem centres on the possibility of storage for prolonged periods. Human semen is now routinely frozen and stored for future use; there appears to be no upper limit to the length of time for which it is safe for frozen storage to continue before use. However the evidence presented to us drew attention to non-medical problems that may arise if frozen gametes or embryos are used after prolonged storage. Serious legal complications may well arise, for example in relation to inheritance and the use or disposal of frozen semen, eggs and embryos. We discuss these problems in the following paragraphs.

10.5 If our recommendations (see 4.22 and 6.8) are accepted donors will have no rights or obligations with regard to their donations when semen or eggs are donated to benefit some other person. The same will apply when semen or eggs are donated for research. The question of ultimate disposal is therefore the responsibility of those storing the material, bearing in mind so far as possible the donor's wishes, if any have been expressed.

10.6 Disposal problems mainly arise when people have stored semen, eggs or embryos for their own personal use. We first consider the case of stored semen and eggs; secondly the position where a couple have stored an embryo. In both, there are good practical reasons for those responsible for the frozen storage of gametes or embryos to keep in regular touch with the man, woman or couple for whom this has been undertaken.

10.7 It seems to us that the only motive for storage would be to make possible the birth of a child at a subsequent date. For example a man might wish to store semen before undergoing surgery, chemotherapy or radiotherapy that is likely to make him sterile, or because he has sustained a spinal cord injury, in the hope that he may father a child by artificial insemination at a later date. Similarly, in the future, a woman might, for example, wish to store healthy eggs if these could be collected before undergoing surgery that might result in the removal of her ovaries. Her hope would be that she might have a child at a future date by IVF. Such men and women might well be only in their teens when their gametes are first stored. Therefore we feel it is unreasonable to put an absolute limit on the length of time for which eggs or semen can be stored. On the other hand it would also be unreasonable and impractical to expect those responsible for storage to maintain all eggs and semen stored indefinitely.

10.8 We believe there should be a system of five yearly reviews. When the reviews are carried out, men and women who have stored semen or eggs can indicate whether they wish storage to continue or whether they have no further use for the gametes and wish them to be destroyed or donated. As a matter of good practice we also suggest that those responsible for storage should consult the individuals who have deposited semen or eggs to ascertain their wishes well in advance of the expiry of the five years. **We recommend that there should be automatic five-yearly reviews of semen and egg deposits. We recommend that legislation provide that where a person dies during the storage period or cannot be traced at a review date the right of use or disposal of his or her frozen gametes should pass to the storage authority.** In this latter situation, as a matter of good practice the storage authority should, in disposing of them, bear in mind any previously expressed wishes in relation to disposal.

10.9 The use by a widow of her dead husband's semen for AIH is a practice which we feel should be actively discouraged. Despite our own views in this matter, (see 4.4) we realise that such requests may occasionally be made. It is obviously essential that there should be some finality for those administering estates of deceased persons since, in such cases posthumous fertilisation could cause real problems of inheritance and succession. Account would have to be taken of issue who might be born years after the death. **We recommend that legislation be introduced to provide that any child born by AIH who was not *in utero* at the date of the death of its father shall be disregarded for the purposes of succession to and inheritance from the latter.**

10.10 We also considered the case where a couple had stored an embryo for their own future use. Such an embryo might exist as a result of IVF when more eggs had been successfully fertilised than were needed for immediate embryo transfer. In this situation embryo storage might be undertaken so that further transfers might be made if the initial IVF treatment proved unsuccessful, or for a subsequent pregnancy, without the need for the woman to undergo further egg recovery. In such cases the couple might very well wish to have more than one child, and we had therefore to bear in mind their need to space pregnancies. At the same time there should in our opinion be a definite time limit set to the storage of embryos both because of the current ignorance of the possible effects of long storage and because of the legal and ethical complications that might arise over disposal of embryos whose parents have died or divorced or otherwise been separated. We believe that, as in the case of semen and eggs, there should be a review after five years of all embryos held and that the maximum time for storage of an embryo should be ten years. **We recommend a maximum of ten years for storage of embryos after which time the right to use or disposal should pass to the storage authority.**

10.11 Until now the law has never had to consider the existence of embryos outside the mother's uterus. The existence of such embryos raises potentially difficult problems as to ownership. The concept of ownership of human embryos seems to us to be undesirable. **We recommend that legislation be enacted to ensure there is no right of ownership in a human embryo.** Nevertheless, the couple who have stored an embryo for their use should be recognised as having rights to the use and disposal of the embryo, although these rights ought to be subject to limitation. The precise nature of that limitation will obviously require careful consideration. We hope the couple will recognise that they have a responsibility to make a firm decision as to the disposal and use of the embryo.

10.12 We consider that the position that may arise in the event of the death of one or both of a couple who have stored an embryo should be clarified. **We therefore recommend that when one of a couple dies the right to use or dispose or any embryo stored by that couple should pass to the survivor.** We make this recommendation notwithstanding our reservations about the possibility of posthumous pregancies. **We recommend that if both die that right should pass to the storage authority.**

10.13 Problems might also arise when, whether in cases of marital breakdown or not, the couple fail to agree how the shared embryo should be used. **We recommend that where there is no agreement between the couple the right to** determine the use or disposal of an embryo should pass to the storage authority as though the ten year period had expired. This recommendation and those in the previous paragraph will require legislation.

10.14 On the question of inheritance and succession we hold that the order in which fertilisation *in vitro* took place should not alter the principle that the first born among siblings in a multiple pregnancy is deemed to be the eldest. The same principle should apply to embryos that have been stored. **We recommend, therefore, that for the purposes of establishing primogeniture the date and time of birth, and not the date of fertilisation, shall be the determining factor.**

10.15 With regard to the possibility of a frozen embryo being transferred to the mother after the death of the father we consider that a similar situation to that which we have recommended in the case of posthumous AIH should apply (see 10.9). **We therefore recommend that legislation be introduced to provide that any child born following IVF, using an embryo that had been frozen and stored, who was not *in utero* at the date of the death of the father shall be disregarded for the purposes of succession to and inheritance from the latter.**

CHAPTER ELEVEN

SCIENTIFIC ISSUES

Human Embryos and Research

11.1 We now turn to the issues arising from the possible use of human embryos for *scientific research*. The question before the Inquiry was whether such research should be allowed. To answer this we found it necessary to look at the very earliest stages of human embryonic development, described in the following paragraphs (11.2 to 11.7).

Early human development

11.2 At fertilisation the egg and sperm unite to become a single cell. The nucleus of this cell contains the chromosomes derived from both parents. This single cell is totipotential, as from it develop all the different types of tissue and organs that make up the human body, as well as the tissues that become the placenta and foetal membranes during intra-uterine development. *In vivo*, fertilisation takes place in the upper portion of the fallopian tube and the fertilised egg then passes down the fallopian tube into the cavity of the uterus over a period of four to five days. At first, when it reaches the cavity of the uterus, it remains free-floating until it begins to attach to the uterine wall at the start of implantation. This is considered to begin on the sixth day following fertilisation. During implantation, which occurs over a period of six to seven days, the embryo enters the endometrium, the lining of the uterus; at the eleventh to thirteenth day after fertilisation, implantation is complete.

11.3 While the fertilised egg is still in the upper portion of the fallopian tube, it begins to divide into first two, then four, then eight, then sixteen smaller cells, and so on by a process called cleavage. At the start of cleavage, in a two or four-cell embryo, each cell retains its totipotential capacity. Thus if separation occurs at the two-cell stage, each may develop to form a separate embryo. Such a separation could lead to identical twins.

11.4 When sixteen or more cells have resulted from cleavage, the cells hang together in a loosely packed configuration, similar to that of a blackberry, called a morula. The morula stage is reached at about the same time as the embryo *in vivo* reaches the uterine cavity. At about the same time a fluid-filled space begins to form in an eccentric position within the substance of the morula. Once this accumulation of fluid has occurred the embryo is described as a blastocyst. Within the blastocyst a thicker section of the cyst wall becomes identifiable as the inner cell mass; it is within the inner cell mass that the embryo proper, eventually to become the foetus, develops. The remaining cells of the thin walled portion of the blastocyst develop to become part of the placenta and foetal membranes. At about the time that the blastocyst begins to implant, a second fluid-filled space, the amniotic cavity, also appears within the inner cell mass. Between the two cystic spaces within the blastocyst, a plate of cells is formed. This is described as the embryonic disc; within it the first recognisable features of the embryo proper will appear.

11.5 The first of these features is the primitive streak, which appears as a heaping-up of cells at one end of the embryonic disc on the fourteenth or fifteenth day after fertilisation. Two primitive streaks may form in a single embryonic disc. This is the latest stage at which identical twins can occur. The primitive streak is the first of several identifiable features which develop in and from the embryonic disc during the succeeding days, a period of very rapid change in the embryonic configuration. By the seventeenth day the neural groove appears and by the twenty-second to twenty-third day this has developed to become the neural folds, which in turn start to fuse and form the recognisable antecedent of the spinal cord.

11.6 Once fertilisation has occurred, the subsequent developmental processes follow one another in a systematic and structured order, leading in turn through cleavage, to the morula, the blastocyst, development of the embryonic disc, and then to identifiable features within the embryonic disc such as the primitive streak, neural folds and neural tube. Until the blastocyst stage has been reached the embryo *in vivo* is unattached, floating first in the fallopian tube and then in the uterine cavity. From the sixth to the twelfth or thirteenth day internal development proceeds within the blastocyst while during the same period implantation is taking place. Both the internal and external processes of development are crucial to the future of the embryo. If the inner cell mass does not form within the blastocyst there is no further embryonic development; while if implantation does not occur the blastocyst is lost at or before the next menstrual period.

11.7 Identical developmental processes are followed by embryos fertilised *in vitro*. In these, following fertilisation, the first cleavage divisions will occur before the embryo is transferred back to the uterus. Thereafter, where implantation takes place, the developmental process will be identical for both *in vitro* and *in vivo* embryos, but there is a very high wastage rate for both as a result of their frequent failure to implant.

The starting point for discussion

11.8 It was the development of IVF that, for the first time, gave rise to the possibility that human embryos might be brought into existence which might have no chance to implant because they were not transferred to a uterus and hence no chance to be born as human beings. This inevitably led to an examination of the moral rights of the embryo.

11.9 Some people hold that if an embryo is human and alive, it follows that it should not be deprived of a chance for development, and therefore it should not be used for research. They would give moral approval to IVF if, and only if, each embryo produced were to be transferred to a uterus. Others, while in no way denying that human embryos are alive, (and they would concede that eggs and sperm are also alive), hold that embryos are not yet human persons and that if it could be decided when an embryo becomes a person, it could also be decided when it might, or might not, be permissible for research to be undertaken. Although the questions of when life or personhood begin appear to be questions of fact susceptible of straightforward answers, we hold that the answers to such questions in fact are complex amalgams of factual and moral judgements. Instead of trying to answer these questions directly we have therefore gone straight to the question of *how it is right to treat the human embryo*. We have considered what status ought to be accorded to the human embryo, and the answer we give must necessarily be in terms of ethical or moral principles.

Defining the limits of research

11.10 We have so far simply spoken of research and given little indication of the scope of this term. We believe that a broad division into two categories can be made. The first, which we term pure research, is aimed at increasing and developing knowledge of the very early stages of the human embryo; the second, applied research, is research with direct diagnostic or therapeutic aims for the human embryo, or for the alleviation of infertility in general. Research aimed at improving IVF techniques would come into this second category. We exclude from the concept of research what we have called new and untried treatment, undertaken during the attempt to alleviate the infertility of a particular patient. We recognise that these distinctions are not absolute. The categories may often overlap, but we feel that they have a certain validity.

Arguments against the use of human embryos

11.11 It is obvious that the central objection to the use of human embryos as research subjects is a fundamental objection, based on moral principles. Put simply, the main argument is that the use of human embryos for research is morally wrong because of the very fact that they are human, and much of the evidence submitted to us strongly supports this. The human embryo is seen as having the same status as a child or an adult, by virtue of its potential for human life. The right to life is held to be the fundamental human right, and the taking of human life on this view is always abhorrent. To take the life of the innocent is an especial moral outrage. The first consequence of this line of argument is that, since an embryo used as a research subject would have no prospect of fulfilling its potential for life, such research should not be permitted.

11.12 Everyone agrees that it is completely unacceptable to make use of a child or an adult as the subject of a research procedure which may cause harm or death. For people who hold the views outlined in 11.11, research on embryos would fall under the same principle. They proceed to argue that since it is unethical to carry out any research, harmful or otherwise, on humans without first obtaining their informed consent, it must be equally unacceptable to carry out research on a human embryo, which by its very nature, cannot give consent.

11.13 In addition to the arguments outlined above, and well represented in the evidence, many people feel an instinctive opposition to research which they see as tampering with the creation of human life. There is widely felt concern at the possibility of unscrupulous scientists meddling with the process of reproduction in order to create hybrids, or to indulge theories of selective breeding and eugenic selection.

11.14 Those who are firmly opposed to research on human embryos recognise that a ban on their use may reduce the volume not only of pure research but also research in potentially beneficial areas, such as the detection and prevention of inherited disorders, or the alleviation of infertility, and that in some areas such a ban would halt research completely. However they argue that the moral principle outweighs any such possible benefits.

Arguments for the use of human embryos

11.15 The evidence showed that the views of those who support the use of human embryos as research subjects cover a wide range. At one end is the proposition that it is only to *human persons* that respect must be accorded. A human embryo cannot be thought of as a person, or even as a potential person. It is simply a collection of cells which, unless it implants in a human uterine environment, has no potential for development. There is no reason therefore to accord these cells any protected status. If useful results can be obtained from research on embryos, then such research should be permitted. We found that the more generally held position, however, is that though the human embryo is entitled to some added measure of respect beyond that accorded to other animal subjects, that respect cannot be absolute, and may be weighed against the benefits arising from research. Although many research studies in embryology and developmental biology can be carried out on animal subjects, and it is possible in many cases to extrapolate these results and findings to man, in certain situations there is no substitute for the use of human embryos. This particularly applies to the study of disorders occurring only in humans, such as Down's syndrome, or for research into the processes of human fertilisation, or perhaps into the specific effect of drugs or toxic substances on human tissue.

The legal position

11.16 We examined the current position of the *in vivo* embryo in law. The human embryo *per se* has no legal status. It is not, under law in the United Kingdom accorded the same status as a child or an adult, and the law does not treat the human embryo as having a right to life. However, there are certain statutory provisions that give some level of protection in various respects. The effect of the Offences Against the Person Act 1861, together with the Abortion Act 1967 (in Scotland the common law as amended by the Abortion Act 1967), is such that abortion is a criminal offence save in the circumstances provided for by the legislation. The Infant Life Preservation Act 1929 (which does not apply in Scotland) has as its purpose the protection of the life of a child capable of being born alive. Under civil law in England and Wales the Congenital Disabilities (Civil Liability) Act 1976 allows, in limited circumstances, damages to be recovered where an embryo or foetus has been injured *in utero* through the negligence of some third person. It is thus accorded a kind of retrospective status where it is born deformed or damaged as a result of injury. This Act does not apply in Scotland or Northern Ireland. The legal position at common law is thought to be similar in Scotland, although the law has yet to be tested. Thus, at present the law provides a measure of protection for the embryo *in vivo*. The remainder of this chapter deals exclusively with the *in vitro* embryo.

11.17 Although, therefore, the law provides a measure of protection for the human embryo *in vivo* it is clear that the human embryo under our definition of the term (1.4) is not, under the present law in the UK accorded the same status as a living child or an adult, nor do we necessarily wish it to be accorded that same status. Nevertheless we were agreed that the embryo of the human species ought to have a special status and that no one should undertake research on human embryos the purposes of which could be achieved by the use of other animals or in some other way. The status of the embryo is a matter of fundamental principle which should be enshrined in legislation. **We recommend that the embryo of the human species should be afforded some protection in law.** We examine below what that protection should be.

11.18 That protection should exist does not entail that this protection may not be waived in certain specific circumstances. Having examined the evidence presented to us about the types of research which might be carried out on human embryos produced *in vitro,* the majority of us[1] hold that such

---

[1] See expression of dissent by Mrs Carriline, Professor Marshall and Mrs Walker.

research should not be totally prohibited. We do not want to see a situation in which human embryos are frivolously or unnecessarily used in research but we are bound to take account of the fact that the advances in the treatment of infertility, which we have discussed in the earlier part of this report, could not have taken place without such research; and that continued research is essential, if advances in treatment and medical knowledge are to continue. A majority of us therefore agreed that research on human embryos should continue. Nevertheless, because of the special status that we accord to the human embryo, such research must be subject to stringent controls and monitoring. Moreover, we would not want any handling or transportation of human embryos *in vitro* to fall outside these controls. **We recommend that research conducted on human *in vitro* embryos and the handling of such embryos should be permitted only under licence. We recommend that any unauthorised use of an *in vitro* embryo would in itself constitute a criminal offence.**[2] We discuss how such controls should be established in Chapter Thirteen. We see these controls as essential to safeguard the public interest and to allay widespread anxiety.

Time limit on keeping embryos alive *in vitro*

11.19 The statutory body which we propose should issue licences for research will have as one of its main functions the regulation of research. First it will have to be assured that no other research material is available (13.11) for the particular project in mind, and second, it will have to limit the length

---

[1] *Aborted embryos*

The focus of this chapter is on the very early human embryo. Almost all of these embryos will result from *in vitro* fertilisation, although some might be obtained from uterine lavage. We are conscious, however, that there are other whole live embryos and foetuses of greater gestational age, which may become available for research following termination of pregnancy. We recognise that both abortion and the Code of Practice contained in the report on "The Use of Fetuses and Fetal Material for Research" (The Peel Report) HMSO 1972 are very much outside our terms of reference. Nevertheless it seems to us totally illogical to propose stringent legislative controls on the use of very early human embryos for research, while there is a less formal mechanism governing the research use of whole live embryos and foetuses of more advanced gestation. Although we understand that these mechanisms have worked well, we consider there is a case for bringing any research that makes use of whole live aborted embryos or foetuses—whether obtained from *in vitro* fertilisation, uterine lavage, or termination of pregnancy—within the sort of legislative framework proposed in this report. We suggest that this be given urgent consideration.

of time for which an embryo can be kept alive *in vitro*. While, as we have seen, the timing of the different stages of development is critical, once the process has begun, there is no particular part of the developmental process that is more important than another; all are part of a continuous process, and unless each stage takes place normally, at the correct time, and in the correct sequence, further development will cease. Thus biologically there is no one single identifiable stage in the development of the embryo beyond which the *in vitro* embryo should not be kept alive. However we agreed that this was an area in which some precise decision must be taken, in order to allay public anxiety.

11.20 The evidence showed a wide range of opinion on this question. One argument put forward may be termed the strictly utilitarian view. This suggests that the ethics of experiments on embryos must be determined by the balance of benefit over harm, or pleasure over pain. Therefore, as long as the embryo is incapable of feeling pain, it is argued that its treatment does not weigh in the balance. According to this argument the time limit for *in vitro* development, and for research on the embryo, could be set either when the first beginnings of the central nervous system can be identified, or when functional activity first occurs. If the former is chosen, this would imply a limit of twenty-two to twenty-three days after fertilisation, when the neural tube begins to close. As to the latter, in the present state of knowledge the onset of central nervous system functional activity could not be used to define accurately the limit to research, because the timing is not known; however, it is generally thought to be considerably later in pregnancy. With either limit, proponents suggest subtracting a few days in order that there would be no possibility of the embryo feeling pain.

11.21 The Royal College of Obstetricians and Gynaecologists suggested that embryos should not be allowed to develop *in vitro* beyond a limit of seventeen days, as this is the point at which early neural development begins. The British Medical Association favoured a limit of fourteen days and a number of groups, including the Medical Research Council and the Royal College of Physicians suggested that the limit should be at the end of the implantation stage. Again, some groups submitting evidence suggested that no embryo which had gone beyond the beginning of the implantation stage should be used for research.

The Inquiry's view

11.22 As we have seen, the objection to using human embryos in research is that each one is a potential human being. One reference point in the development of the human individual is the formation of the primitive streak (11.5). Most authorities put this at about fifteen days after fertilisation. This marks the beginning of individual development of the embryo. Taking such a time limit is consonant with the views of those who favour the end of the implantation stage as a limit. We have therefore regarded an earlier date than this as a desirable end-point for research. **We accordingly recommend that no live human embryo derived from *in vitro* fertilisation, whether frozen or unfrozen, may be kept alive, if not transferred to a woman, beyond fourteen days after fertilisation, nor may it be used as a research subject beyond fourteen days after fertilisation. This fourteen day period does not include any time during which the embryo may have been frozen. We further recommend that it shall be a criminal offence to handle or to use as a research subject any live human embryo derived from *in vitro* fertilisation beyond that limit. We recommend that no embryo which has been used for research should be transferred to a woman.**

11.23 A further question on which the licensing body will have to be satisfied is the origin of the embryos to be used. There is a number of possible sources of human embryos for research use. First, as we pointed out in Chapter Five, current IVF procedures often result in the production of a number of "spare" embryos that will not be transferred to a woman and these, if they are not needed for treatment purposes, could be used as research subjects. Second, clearly it is also possible to produce embryos *in vitro*, using donated eggs and semen, with the sole intention of using them for research. Third, a possible source would be embryos which happened to be produced during the course of research concentrating on, for example the fertilising capacity of human eggs or semen, but where the primary aim of that research is not to bring embryos into existence.

11.24 We are satisfied that "spare" embryos may be used as subjects for research; **and we recommend accordingly a need to obtain *consent* to the method of use or disposal of spare embryos. We recommend that as a matter of**

good practice no research should be carried out on a spare embryo without the informed consent of the couple for whom that embryo was generated, whenever this is possible.

11.25 The problem discussed in the following paragraphs was a very difficult one for the Inquiry to resolve and members gave it a great deal of thought over an extended period. Some members although they agree that research on spare embryos may legitimately be undertaken, see a clear moral distinction between the research use of embryos available by chance, which were not needed for the purposes of treatment, and on the other hand the generation of embryos brought into being for the purposes of research alone and where there is no question of their being transferred to a woman. And this includes embryos which come into existence as a by-product of research on fertilisation (see 11.23). These members argue that it cannot be consonant with the special status that the Inquiry as a whole has agreed should be afforded to the human embryo, to cause it to exist, yet to allow it no possibility of implantation. Similarly others argue that it is fertilisation itself that is unique and it ought not to be undertaken when there is no chance whatever that the potential for human development will be fulfilled.

11.26 All members who are opposed to the deliberate gene-ration of embryos for research accept that this might slow down the pace of research and that not every kind of research could be carried out using only embryos which were adventitiously available. Despite the fact that the research in question would be mainly for the alleviation of infertility and the prevention of hereditary disease, they adhere to the view that, whatever the handicap to scientific progress, it would be morally wrong to bring human embryos into being solely for the purpose of research.

11.27 There is a further argument that if it is once thought permissible to allow embryos to come into being with the sole intention that they be used for research, this would open the way for an ever-increasing use of human embryos for routine and less valid research, whatever may have been the original intention of regulation. Once a foot is set on the "slippery slope" of deliberate creation of embryos, no end can be set to the dangers. Nevertheless, the argument runs, research on embryos may be justified, provided that the embryos used as subjects of research were brought into being, not primarily for research, but in order to alleviate a particular case of infertility. This argument in part rests on the doctrine known to philosophers as "double effect": an act which would be wrong if chosen for its own sake may be justified if it occurs as a by-product of some other, well-intentioned act. According to this view, therefore, there would be no general acceptance of research on embryos, but acceptance only in the limited circumstance of the existence of "spare" embryos. Those who hold this view would argue that it would be preferable on moral grounds that there should be no research on embryos rather than research regardless of the circumstances in which the embryos were brought into being.

11.28 Other members did not make the same distinction between spare and deliberately generated embryos. They argue that if research on human embryos is to be permitted at all, it makes no difference whether these embryos happen to be available or were brought into existence for the sake of research. In neither case would these embryos have a potential for life, because in neither case were they to be transferred to a uterus. Further, in both cases, research would be subject to the limitations outlined above and the moral status of the embryo would be the same, and subject to the same fourteen day limitation.

11.29 Members who hold this view give a great deal of weight to the consideration that to prohibit the generation of embryos specifically for research would severely curtail the range and scientific validity of research on human embryos, and in some fields would effectively preclude it entirely. In addition, even if some gametes were donated for research purposes, it would not be possible to undertake any research on the process of fertilisation itself using human eggs and sperm since this process would necessarily result in some cases in the generation of an embryo. Research on the fertilisation of eggs stored by freezing is essential if there is ever to be the possibility that frozen eggs may be used in infertility treatment; and the use of frozen eggs, if the technique could be developed, would raise fewer ethical problems than the freezing of embryos. A further argument for the generation of embryos for research is that as the techniques of freezing become more successful there would be fewer spare embryos available for research. For couples would probably prefer to freeze any embryos which could not be used immediately in an IVF treatment for use either if the initial embryo transfer were unsuccessful, or for a subsequent pregnancy. Moreover it is argued that spare embryos are not necessarily ideal material for research. Inevitably and quite rightly, those embryos that are developing best are replaced in the mother, and the "spares" tend to be less good. This could well affect the findings of any research project.

11.30 Members of the Inquiry who subscribed to the view (11.24) that research on spare embryos should be permitted were nevertheless divided[1] on the question whether research should be permitted on embryos brought into existence specifically for that purpose or coming into existence as a result of other research. However, we are nevertheless agreed that the issue is of such importance that it should be controlled by legislation, and not left to the discretion of the licensing body. Despite our division on this point, a majority of us **recommend that the legislation should provide that research may be carried out on any embryo resulting from *in vitro* fertilisation, whatever its provenance, up to the end of the fourteenth day after fertilisation, but subject to all other restrictions as may be imposed by the licensing body.**

[1] See expression of dissent by T S G Baker, Professor Dyson, Mrs Edwards and Doctor Greengross.

CHAPTER TWELVE

POSSIBLE FUTURE DEVELOPMENTS IN RESEARCH

12.1 There is a number of specific techniques and procedures involving the use of human embryos which have caused much public anxiety. Many of these have not yet reached the stage where they are practical possibilities. We believe that our recommendations for the regulation of research will allay much of that anxiety, as it will be the duty of the proposed licensing body (13.3) to keep these and other new techniques under constant review; indeed, in some instances our proposals will preclude certain developments altogether. It is important, however, to consider whether further restrictions are required, although it must be borne in mind that we cannot foresee all possible developments.

A current technique that requires regulation: Trans-species fertilisation

12.2 A test in which human sperm may fertilise hamster eggs is already used in the investigation of male subfertility. Men whose sperm will fertilise a specially treated hamster egg may eventually father a child, whereas those whose sperm will not are probably infertile. Although in the hamster test any resulting embryo does not develop beyond the two cell stage, it is possible that other similar forms of trans-species fertilisation tests could be developed. Unlike the hamster test, such tests might result in an embryo which might develop for a considerable period of time. Both the hamster tests and the possibility of other trans-species fertilisations, carried out either diagnostically or as part of a research project, have caused public concern about the prospect of developing hybrid half-human creatures.

12.3 We take the view that trans-species fertilisation when undertaken as part of a recognised programme for alleviating infertility, or in the assessment or diagnosis of subfertility, is an acceptable procedure, subject to certain safeguards. Since the object is to assess fertilising capacity, we see no reason why any resultant embryo should be allowed to survive beyond the two-cell stage. **We recommend that where trans-species fertilisation is used as part of a recognised programme for alleviating infertility or in the assessment or diagnosis of subfertility it should be subject to licence and that a condition of granting such a licence should be that the development of any resultant hybrid should be terminated at the two cell stage. Any unlicensed use of trans-species fertilisation involving human gametes should be a criminal offence.**

Techniques that might be developed in the future

12.4 There is a number of other techniques which, although their development would be some way in the future, have been a subject of speculation and have aroused considerable interest.

Use of human embryos for testing drugs etc

12.5 It has been suggested that human embryos could be used to test the effects of newly developed drugs or other substances that may possibly be toxic or cause abnormalities. This is an area that causes deep concern because of the possibility of mass production of *in vitro* embryos, perhaps on a commercial basis, for these purposes. We feel very strongly that the routine testing of drugs on human embryos is not an acceptable area of research because this would require the manufacture of large numbers of embryos. We concluded however that there may be very particular circumstances where the testing of such substances on a very small scale may be justifiable.

12.6 In our view any research project in this area would have to be subject to very close scrutiny and it would rest with the proposed licensing body (13.3) to come to a decision according to the merits of each particular research project submitted to it.

Ectogenesis

12.7 It has been suggested that in the long term further development of current techniques could result in the maintenance of developing embryos in an artificial environment (ectogenesis) for progressively longer periods with the ultimate aim of creating a child entirely *in vitro*. This technique, it is argued, would make it possible to study in detail normal and abnormal human development at the embryonic and foetal stages.

12.8 We appreciate why the possibility of such a technique arouses so much anxiety. There are however two points to make about this. First, such developments are well into the future, certainly beyond the time horizon within which this Inquiry feels it can predict. Secondly, our recommendation is that the growing of a human embryo *in vitro* beyond fourteen days should be a criminal offence.

Gestation of human embryos in other species

12.9 Another cause for concern is the suggestion that a human embryo might be transferred to the uterus of another species for gestation. While the available animal work does not suggest that it is at all likely that human embryos could be nurtured in the uterus of another species, the possibility that such an experiment might be attempted must be recognised. **We recommend that the placing of a human embryo in the uterus of another species for gestation should be a criminal offence.**

Parthenogenesis

12.10 This term is used to describe the reproductive process whereby a gamete develops into a new individual without fertilisation. This form of reproduction occurs in some invertebrate species and plants. Although it is known that the application of some substances, for example, alcohol, to an unfertilised mammalian egg can induce the egg to undergo some initial development, we consider that there is no possibility at present of inducing parthenogenesis, or "virgin birth" as it is commonly known, in humans, and indeed we do not believe such a development will take place in the foreseeable future.

Cloning

12.11 Cloning is the production of two or more genetically identical individuals. Human identical twins are the result of natural cloning. One method of achieving cloning would be by division of the embryo at a very early stage of development so that identical genetic material is passed on to each of the separate portions. Thus all members of a clone have an identical genetic constitution. This type of cloning has been used successfully on other species but, to the best of our knowledge, has not been carried out artificially on human embryos.

Embryonic biopsy

12.12 It has been suggested that a similar technique to cloning could be used to investigate the chromosomal structure of embryos fertilised *in vitro* by a couple who have a high chance of procreating an abnormal child. After *in vitro* fertilisation, the embryo would be allowed to develop until it was possible to remove one or more cells without putting at risk the subsequent development of the embryo. This technique is termed embryonic biopsy. The cells of the biopsy would be allowed to continue to develop while the rest of the embryo would be frozen. Once it was possible to determine from the biopsy whether the embryo was free of the abnormality for which it was being tested, a decision could be taken as to whether to thaw the fozen embryo and to transfer it to the mother's uterus.

12.13 It is difficult to estimate how likely it is that embryonic biopsy will be developed as a diagnostic technique in the near future. It has the advantage over other techniques such as chorion biopsy (9.7) that may be used for the early diagnosis of abnormalities, in that it may be carried out before the embryo is transferred and so before there is a pregnancy, thus avoiding the difficult decision for the parents of whether to seek a termination where abnormality is detected. However, it has the disadvantage that it requires the use of IVF. Given the present relatively low success rates for pregnancy following IVF, it is unlikely that embryonic biopsy will become a feasible method of detecting abnormal embryos for some considerable time.

Nucleus substitution

12.14 Another technique, which has sometimes been referred to as cloning, but which may be more accurately described as nucleus substitution would raise more fundamental questions. These would occur if it became possible to remove the nucleus from a fertilised human egg and, without detriment to its subsequent development, replace it with the nucleus taken from an adult human. This process would open the way for the creation of "carbon copy clones". It has been suggested that one day it might be possible to produce immunologically identical organs for transplantation purposes to replace a diseased organ, for example a kidney. The cloned replacement organ would be grown in an embryo in which the nucleus had been replaced by one taken from the person for whom the replacement organ was intended.

Prevention of genetic defects

12.15 If it should become possible to identify at a very early stage of embryonic development certain genetic defects; and to insert a replacement gene which will remedy the defect, a genetically normal embryo could be created. It is argued that this would provide the means to prevent certain genetic diseases.

12.16 Public anxiety about these techniques centres, not so much on their possible therapeutic use, but on the idea of the deliberate creation of human beings with specific characteristics. This has overtones of selective breeding. We regard such techniques as purely speculative but believe that any developments in these fields are precluded by the controls we have already recommended. We would however go further. **We recommend that the proposed licensing body promulgates guidance on what types of research, apart from those precluded by law, would be unlikely to be considered ethically acceptable in any circumstances and therefore would not be licensed.** We envisage this guidance being reviewed from time to time to take account of both changes in scientific knowledge and changes in public attitudes.

CHAPTER THIRTEEN

REGULATING INFERTILITY SERVICES AND RESEARCH

13.1 Public concern about the techniques we have discussed needs to be reflected in public policy. We believe that all the techniques require active regulation and monitoring, even though, as we realise, such restrictions may be regarded by some as infringing clinical or academic freedom. It is not our intention to interfere with the duty of the doctor to exercise clinical judgement in treating patients. Indeed we accept and expect the doctor to be the person who makes the final decision about whether a treatment is likely to succeed, and whether it should be used. Similarly we accept that scientists must not be unduly restricted in pursuing their research interests especially when this may produce direct therapeutic benefits.

13.2 But doctors and scientists work within the moral and legal framework determined by society. They do not and should not depart radically from that framework. Our intention is that activities which have evolved in an unstructured and unmonitored way should be placed on a properly organised basis, within a framework broadly acceptable to society. The interests of those directly concerned, as well as those of society in general, demand that certain legal and ethical safeguards should be applied.

13.3 The protection of the public, which we see as the primary objective of regulation, demands the existence of an authority independent of Government, health authorities, or research institutions. The authority should be specifically charged with the responsibility to regulate and monitor practice in relation to those sensitive areas which raise fundamental ethical questions. **We therefore recommend the establishment of a new statutory licensing authority to regulate both research and those infertility services which we have recommended should be subject to control.**

13.4 Although we do not see it as our function to specify the precise size and detailed composition of the new body, there are some general points which we would like to make. The new body will need access to expert medical and scientific advice. We would therefore envisage a significant representation of scientific and medical interests among the membership. It would also need to have members experienced in the organisation and provision of services. However, this is not exclusively, or even primarily, a medical or scientific body. It is concerned essentially with broader matters and with the protection of the public interest. If the public is to have confidence that this is an independent body, which is not to be unduly influenced by sectional interests, its membership must be wide-ranging and in particular the lay interests should be well represented. **We recommend that there should be substantial lay representation on the statutory authority to regulate research and infertility services and that the chairman must be a lay person.**

Functions of the new body

13.5 We envisage the new body having two distinct functions, one advisory and one executive. We believe it should issue general guidance, to those working in the field, on good practice in infertility service provision and on the types of research which, without prejudice to its view of any individual project, it finds broadly ethically acceptable. It should also offer advice to Government on specific issues as they arise, and be available for Ministers to consult for specific guidance. As part of its responsibility to protect the public interest, it should publish and present to Parliament, an Annual Report, setting out the facilities for infertility treatment currently licensed and the research currently in progress, its purpose and scope, including an indication of the number of embryos being used, and their type, so that this knowledge may be publicly available.

13.6 Its executive function would be twofold: to grant licences to those wishing to offer the kinds of infertility treatment we have discussed, whether in the NHS or in the private sector; and to grant licences to researchers wishing to work with human gametes and embryos. The licensing body would be supported by an inspectorate, who would undertake regular inspections of premises where such work was carried out, to ensure that licence holders were keeping to the terms of their licences and meeting the prescribed conditions. We do not see it as our function to specify in detail the criteria for granting a licence but there are certain controls which we believe should be imposed. These are discussed in the paragraphs that follow.

Licensing of infertility services

13.7 **We recommend that all practitioners offering the services that we have recommended should only be provided under licence, and all premises used as part of any such provision, including the provision of fresh semen and banks for the storage of frozen human eggs, semen and embryos should be licensed by the licensing body.**

13.8 Licensed infertility services should be run by a qualified medical practitioner with appropriately qualified supporting staff and adequate facilities. We have given some thought to whether there is a need for special training for infertility services, but have concluded that training, as in other spheres of medicine, should be the responsibility of the appropriate professional bodies. The existence of screening arrangements sufficient to meet a centrally determined standard must be one of the criteria for granting a licence. Once donors have been selected there must be satisfactory arrangements for handling of semen and eggs to ensure that the quality of both is satisfactory and remains so. Any frozen semen or eggs must be properly identifiable throughout the time they are stored, so that there is no danger of confusion. The licensing body should therefore concern itself with these aspects of quality control.

13.9 We would also like the licensing body to consider what follow-up of children born as a result of the new techniques may be needed. We recognise that there are those who believe that any systematic follow-up or research studies would be unduly intrusive, since they would mark out the children and families as in some way different. On the other hand it is argued that only through such studies will it be possible to assess the long-term consequences, both physical, psychological and developmental of the use of these techniques. It is further argued that it is particularly important as a reassurance to prospective parents, to confirm the present understanding that there are no additional risks of abnormality from their use. There is also the question as to whether, as a basis for such follow-up studies, there should be a centrally-maintained record of all births. Such a register would enable children on reaching their majority to check whether they were born as a result of any of the new techniques and to discover the information to which they are entitled (see 4.21, 6.6 and 7.7). We recognise the difficulties in establishing such a register, in terms of ensuring completeness, and in relation to confidentiality; for these reasons we have not seen it as part of our remit to make firm proposals. Nonetheless, we see the whole area of follow-up activity as in need of urgent consideration and **recommend that the licensing body be asked to consider the need for follow-up studies of children born as a result of the new techniques, including consideration of the need for a centrally maintained register of such births.**

Research Licences

13.10 Research projects will be capable of being licensed so long as they do not infringe the legislative restrictions we have recommended in Chapter Eleven. In order, therefore, to tighten the controls, licences should be granted for individual projects, to expire on the completion of that project. They should be granted to an individual or institution only for specified research in this field. In addition there should be a named licence holder who takes overall responsibility for the project. He or she would be responsible for notifying the licensing authority of the names of any support staff who would be working on the project and who might, at some stage, handle human gametes or embryos.

13.11 In applying for a licence, an applicant would be obliged to indicate clearly the objectives of the research, and why these cannot be achieved by means that do not involve the use, or generation of human embryos. The applicant should be required to indicate the approximate number of embryos to be used, the source of the embryos and the duration of the project, including for how many days embryos would be maintained and how they would be disposed of at the end of that period. The application would have to indicate what records would be maintained and these would have to be available to the inspectorate so that they can be sure that the terms of the licence have been observed. The licensing body should establish that the applicant possesses appropriate qualifications and experience for the work he or she wishes to undertake and that the work is supported by peer review undertaken by appropriate academic referees.

13.12 The new body should have no function in relation to the funding of research. It is to be concerned only with ethical and licensing matters. We do not therefore wish to set guidelines on whether an applicant for a licence should be required to seek funding either before obtaining a licence, or after doing so, or indeed to make simultaneous applications for a licence and for funding. However we consider it crucial that any applicant should have first obtained clearance from the ethical body responsible for such matters in the institution in which he or she wishes to carry out research work before submitting applications. We see this local ethical clearance as a necessary, but not in itself sufficient, requirement for the granting of a licence.

Sale of human gametes and embryos

13.13 There is one further area where we see a role for a licensing body. It has been suggested that if the demand for human gametes and embryos, for either treatment or for research, increased, there could be a risk of commercial exploitation and of an export and import trade. We would see this as undesirable. On the other hand we can foresee situations where the supply of human gametes or embryos might reasonably involve some commercial transaction, for example if a licensed semen bank was asked to supply specimens to a distant part of the country which would involve them in considerable costs of transportation, we see no reason why they should not seek reimbursement of expenses. Thus a complete prohibition on the purchase or sale of such material would be inappropriate. A balance has to be struck and therefore **we recommend that the sale or purchase of human gametes or embryos should be permitted only under licence from, and subject to, conditions prescribed by the licensing body and therefore unauthorised sale or purchase should be made a criminal offence.**

Conclusion

13.14 Throughout this report, as well as in the particular matter of the licensing body, we have made no attempt to cost provision. We have aimed throughout to concentrate on principles rather than on details. We have, however, tried to distinguish between the areas where legislation is needed and those within which guidance must come from sources other than Parliament, or where general attitudes must be changed. But of all the recommendations we have made, by far the most urgent is the recommendation that a statutory body should be established, within whose powers would fall the licensing and monitoring of provision for infertility treatment and of research on the human embryo. None of our other recommendations can have any practical impact until such a body is set up.

LIST OF RECOMMENDATIONS

We recommend that:

A. The licensing body and its functions

1. A new statutory licensing authority be established to regulate both research and those infertility services which we have recommended should be subject to control.   13.3

2. There should be substantial lay representation on the statutory authority to regulate research and infertility services and that the chairman must be a lay person.   13.4

3. All practitioners offering the services we have recommended should only be provided under licence, and all premises used as part of any such provision, including the provision of fresh semen and banks for the storage of frozen human eggs, semen and embryos should be licensed by the licensing body.   13.7

4. AID should be available on a properly organised basis and subject to the licensing arrangements described in Chapter Thirteen, to those infertile couples for whom it might be appropriate. The provision of AID services without a licence for the purpose should be an offence.   4.16

5. The service of IVF should continue to be available subject to the same type of licensing and inspection as we have recommended with regard to the regulation of AID (see Chapter Four)   5.10

6. Egg donation be accepted as a recognised technique in the treatment of infertility subject to the same type of licensing and controls as we have recommended for the regulation of AID and IVF.   6.6

7. The form of embryo donation involving donated semen and egg which are brought together *in vitro* be accepted as a treatment for infertility, subject to the same type of licensing and controls as we have recommended with regard to the regulation of AID, IVF and egg donation.   7.4

8. The technique of embryo donation by lavage should not be used at the present time. 7.5

9. The use of frozen eggs in therapeutic procedures should not be undertaken until research has shown that no unacceptable risk is involved. This will be a matter for review by the licensing body. 10.2

10. The clinical use of frozen embryos may continue to be developed under review by the licensing body. 10.3

11. Research conducted on human *in vitro* embryos and the handling of such embryos should be permitted only under licence. 11.8

12. No live human embryo derived from *in vitro* fertilisation, whether frozen or unfrozen, may be kept alive, if not transferred to a woman beyond fourteen days after fertilisation, nor may it be used as a research subject beyond fourteen days after fertilisation. This fourteen day period does not include any time during which the embryo may have been frozen. 11.22

13. Consent be obtained as to the method of use or disposal of spare embryos. 11.24

14. As a matter of good practice no research should be carried out on a spare embryo without the informed consent of the couple for whom the embryo was generated, whenever this is possible. 11.24

15. Where trans-species fertilisation is used as part of a recognised programme for alleviating infertility or in the assessment or diagnosis of sub-fertility it should be subject to licence and that a condition of granting such a licence should be that the development of any resultant hybrid should be terminated at the two cell stage. 12.3

16. The licensing body be asked to consider the need for follow-up studies of children born as a result of the new techniques, including consideration of the need for a centrally maintained register of such births. 13.9

17. The sale or purchase of human gametes or embryos should be permitted only under licence from, and subject to, conditions prescribed by the licensing body. 13.13

B. Principles of provision

18. As a matter of good practice any third party donating gametes for infertility treatment should be unknown to the couple before, during and after the treatment, and equally the third party should not know the identity of the couple being helped. 3.2

19. Counselling should be available to all infertile couples and third parties at any stage of the treatment, both as an integral part of NHS provision and in the private sector. 3.4

20. On reaching the age of eighteen the child should have access to the basic information about the donor's ethnic origin and genetic health and that legislation be enacted — to provide the right of access to this. 4.21

21. In the case of more specialised forms of infertility treatment the consent in writing of both partners should be obtained, wherever possible, before treatment is begun, as a matter of good practice. Any written consent should be obtained on an appropriate consent form. 4.21

22. The formal consent in writing by both partners should, as a matter of good practice, always be obtained before AID treatment begins. A consent form should be used and thoroughly explained to both partners. 4.23

23. For the present, there should be a limit of ten children who can be fathered by one donor. 4.26

24. In cases where consultants decline to provide treatment they should always give the patient a full explanation of the reasons. 2.13

25. The NHS numbers of all donors be checked by the clinics where they make their donations against a new centrally maintained list of NHS numbers of existing donors, which is to be held separately from the NHS donor register. 4.26

26. There should be a gradual move towards a system where semen donors should be given only their expenses. 4.27

27. In relation to egg donation the principles of good practice we have already considered in relation to other techniques should apply, including the anonymity of the donor, limitation of the number of children born from the eggs of any one donor to ten, openness with the child about his genetic origins, the availability of counselling for all parties and informed consent.   6.6

28. It should be accepted practice to offer donated gametes and embryos to those at risk of transmitting hereditary disorders.   9.3

29. All types of "do-it-yourself" sex selection kits should be brought within the ambit of control provided by the Medicines Act with the aim of ensuring that such products are safe, efficacious and of an acceptable standard for use.   9.12

30. The use of frozen semen in artificial insemination should continue.   10.1

31. There should be automatic five-yearly reviews of semen and egg deposits.   10.8

32. There should be a maximum of ten years for the storage of embryos after which time the right to use or disposal should pass to the storage authority.   10.10

33. When one of a couple dies the right to use or dispose of any embryo stored by that couple should pass to the survivor. If both die that right should pass to the storage authority.   10.12

34. Where there is no agreement between the couple the right to determine the use or disposal of an embryo should pass to the storage authority as though the ten year period had expired.   10.13

C. Service provision
35. Funding should be made available for the collection of adequate statistics on infertility and infertility services.   2.14

36. Each health authority should review its facilities for the investigation and treatment of infertility and consider the establishment, separate from routine gynaecology, of a specialist infertility clinic with close working relationships with specialist units, including genetic counselling services, at regional and supra-regional level. 2.16

37. Where it is not possible to have a separate clinic, infertility patients should be seen separately from other types of gynaecological patient, wherever possible. 2.16

38. The establishment of a working group at national level made up of central health departments, health authorities and those working in infertility, to draw up detailed guidance on the organisation of services. 2.17

39. Consideration be given to the inclusion of plans for infertility services as part of the next round of health authority strategic plans. 2.18

40. IVF should continue to be available within the NHS. 5.10

41. One of the first tasks of the working group, whose establishment we recommend in 2.17, should be to consider how best an IVF service can be organised within the NHS. 5.11

D. Legal limits on research

42. The embryo of the human species should be afforded some protection in law. 11.17

43. Any unauthorised use of an *in vitro* embryo would in itself constitute a criminal offence. 11.18

44. Legislation should provide that research may be carried out on any embryo resulting from *in vitro* fertilisation, whatever its provenance, up to the end of the fourteenth day after fertilisation, but subject to all other restrictions as may be imposed by the licensing body. 11.30

45. It shall be a criminal offence to handle or to use as a research subject any live human embryo derived from *in vitro* fertilisation beyond that limit (ie fourteen days after fertilisation).   11.22

46. No embryo which has been used for research should be transferred to a woman.   11.22

47. Any unlicensed use of trans-species fertilisation involving human gametes should be a criminal offence.   12.3

48. The placing of a human embryo in the uterus of another species for gestation should be a criminal offence.   12.9

49. The proposed licensing body promulgates guidance on what types of research, apart from those precluded by law, would be unlikely to be considered ethically acceptable in any circumstances and therefore would not be licenced.   12.16

50. Unauthorised sale or purchase of human gametes or embryos should be made a criminal offence.   13.13

E. Legal changes

51. The AID child should in law be treated as the legitimate child of its mother and her husband, where they have both consented to the treatment.   4.17

52. A change in the law so that the semen donor will have no parental rights or duties in relation to the child.   4.22

53. Following the English Law Commission, that it should be presumed that the husband has consented to AID, unless the contrary is proved.   4.24

54. The law should be changed so as to permit the husband to be registered as the father, (subject to 4.17).   4.25

55. Legislation should provide that when a child is born to a woman following donation of another's egg the woman giving birth should, for all purposes, be regarded in law as the mother of that child, and that the egg donor should have no rights or obligations in respect of the child.   6.8

56. The legislation proposed in 4.25 and 6.8 should cover children born following embryo donation. (see recommendations 53 and 54) 7.6

57. Legislation should be introduced to render criminal the creation or the operation in the United Kingdom of agencies whose purposes include the recruitment of women for surrogate pregnancy or making arrangements for individuals or couples who wish to utilise the services of a carrying mother; such legislation should be wide enough to include both profit and non-profit making organisations. 8.18

58. Legislation should be sufficiently wide enough to render criminally liable the actions of professionals and others who knowingly assist in the establishment of a surrogate pregnancy. 8.18

59. It be provided by statute that all surrogacy agreements are illegal contracts and therefore unenforceable in the courts. 8.19

60. Legislation should provide that where a person dies during the storage period or cannot be traced at a review date the right of use or disposal of his or her frozen gametes should pass to the storage authority. 10.8

61. Legislation be introduced to provide that any child born by AIH who was not *in utero* at the date of the death of its father shall be disregarded for the purposes of succession to and inheritance from the latter. 10.9

62. Legislation be enacted to ensure there is no right of ownership in a human embryo. 10.11

63. For the purposes of establishing primogeniture the date and time of birth and not the date of fertilisation shall be the determining factor. 10.14

64. Legislation be introduced to provide that any child born following IVF, using an embryo that had been frozen and stored, who was not *in utero* at the date of the death of the father shall be disregarded for the purposes of succession to and inheritance from the latter. 10.15

EXPRESSION OF DISSENT: A. SURROGACY

1. In the following paragraphs we express dissent from some of the views of the Inquiry on the question of surrogacy. There are, we hold, rare occasions when surrogacy could be beneficial to couples as a last resort. On those occasions gynaecologists should not be denied the option of suggesting surrogacy to their patients. In the best interests of all concerned, however, and particularly in the best interests of the child that may ensue, we think that stringent care and control is necessary. We recommend that the licensing authority proposed in Chapter Thirteen should include surrogacy within its terms of reference, and that any non-profit making agency that wished to assist in making surrogacy arrangements would have to be licensed by the authority.

2. We wish to make it clear that we share with our colleagues many of the concerns expressed in Chapter Eight. The practice of surrogacy could lead to serious problems, and we do not wish to deny these problems. Equally we regard it as of immense importance that people considering getting involved in surrogacy, in whatever way, should be fully aware of the complications that could ensue. We concur with paragraphs 8.1 to 8.16 as a fair summary of these issues. We begin to part company with our colleagues however in paragraphs 8.17 to 8.19 as the Inquiry's view is spelt out.

3. Even in these paragraphs there is much common ground. We go along entirely with our colleagues in our disapproval of surrogacy for convenience. We also agree that the criminal law should be brought in to prevent the operation of profit making agencies in this field, although our reasons for this are somewhat different from those of our colleagues. In our view the question of exploitation of the surrogate mother, or the treating of her as a means to other people's ends, is not as clear cut a moral issue as our colleagues assert. On the other hand we hold firmly that the very difficult personal, legal and social issues raised by surrogacy lie close to those raised in adoption and fostering and hence that there should be no place for commercial operations just as there is no place for commercial adopting agencies.

4. Our disagreement with our colleagues becomes most marked in paragraphs 8.18 and 8.19. Whatever we as an Inquiry may recommend, the demand for surrogacy in one form or another will continue, and possibly even grow. Some of this demand might well be frivolous or misplaced, but there are undoubtedly couples who, for the medical reasons enunciated in paragraph 8.2, will seek surrogacy as a last resort. Our colleagues, by their recommendation in paragraph 8.18 would prevent gynaecologists from offering any form of assistance to such couples to achieve a surrogate pregnancy. As a consequence couples may give up any hope of a child, may take further risks such as of more miscarriages, or may decide to venture into some sort of "do-it-yourself" arrangement. The latter possibility—that couples are driven into making their own arrangements—is particularly unsatisfactory. These arrangements would be unsupported by medical and counselling services and would lack the anonymity that the Inquiry has recommended in paragraph 3.2 to protect all parties in infertility treatments from legal and emotional complications.

5. Having considered the risks on both sides of a finely balanced argument we have come to the conclusion that it would be a mistake to close the door completely on surrogacy being offered as a treatment for childlessness. We are concerned, however, about the way in which it might be offered. We believe that the licensing authority proposed in Chapter Thirteen should include surrogacy within its remit. The authority would have the power to license an agency or agencies to make arrangements for surrogacy. These arrangements would include the matching of commissioning parents with surrogate mothers, and the provision of adequate counselling to ensure that the legal and personal complications of surrogacy were fully understood. The only agencies which could be licensed would be those in which child-caring skills were well represented and in which there was no commercial motive. Thus adoption and fostering agencies or some new agency, similarly staffed and run, could be appropriate candidates for licensing. We are not suggesting that the licensing authority establish an agency, only if one is proposed it be empowered to consider its application. Access to a licensed agency could only be by referral from a consultant gynaecologist.

6. The presence of a licensed agency should not in our opinion render illegal any surrogacy arrangements that did not

use the agency, as it would clearly be undesirable that a child's conception and birth should have any taint of illegality attached to it. On the other hand anyone (including a medical practitioner) who made surrogacy arrangements for a couple and who was not licensed to do so would be committing an offence, regardless of whether they were acting for profit.

7. We recognise the difficulties in the way of the commissioning couple acquiring parental status (paragraphs 8.8 and 8.9). We believe that if steps are taken to regularise surrogacy through licensing, some form of adoption procedure must be open to couples. Under present law money may not change hands in the process of adoption. Nevertheless, most surrogate mothers would expect payment for their services. In our opinion payments to a surrogate mother should not be a barrier to the child being adopted by the commissioning couple.

8. If our proposals are accepted, we believe that it would be inappropriate for steps to be taken to provide that all surrogacy agreements are illegal contracts (paragraph 8.19). For the time being the Courts should be free to consider individual cases on their own merits if they so choose.

9. We do not believe that public opinion is yet fully formed on the question of surrogacy, which has burst into prominence only in the last year or so. Thus we think it is too early to take a final decision one way or the other. We wish to have the opportunity in the next few years to see what the demand is, whether an agency is prepared to come forward to satisfy it, and whether the consequences are generally acceptable or not. We simply ask that the door be left slightly ajar so that surrogacy can be more effectively assessed.

Wendy Greengross

David Davies

EXPRESSION OF DISSENT: B. USE OF HUMAN EMBRYOS IN RESEARCH

1. We have signed the main report subject to our reservations the reasons for which are set out below on the recommendation in paragraph 18 of Chapter Eleven, from which we dissent. We agree with our colleagues that the embryo of the human species has a special status (11.17) but differ from them as to what this implies.

When does life begin?

2. Public concern about the embryo which led to the establishment of this Inquiry is often expressed in the form of the question, "When does life begin?" This cannot be answered in a simple fashion. An ovum is a living cell as is a spermatozoon; both can be properly described as alive. The cluster of cells which is the embryo is likewise alive. But this is not what people are really ʳ ᵇⁱⁿg. Their real question is "When does the human persɔɳ ɔome into existence?" This cannot be answered in a simple fashion either. The beginning of a person is not a question of fact but of decision made in the light of moral principles. The question must therefore be refined still further. It thus becomes "At what stage of development should the status of a person be accorded to an embryo of the human species?" Different people answer this question in different ways. Some say at fertilisation, others at implantation, yet others at a still later stage of development. Scientific observation and philosophical and theological reflection can illuminate the question but they cannot answer it.

The special status of the embryo

3. The special status of the human embryo and the protection to be afforded to it by law do not in our view depend upon the decision as to when it becomes a person. Clearly, once that status has been accorded all moral principles and legal enactments which relate to persons will apply. But before that point has been reached the embryo has a special status because of its potential for development to a stage at which everyone would accord it the status of a human person. It is in our view wrong to create something with the potential for becoming a human person and then deliberately to destroy it.

We therefore recommend that nothing should be done that would reduce the chance of successful implantation of the embryo.

4. It may be argued that the ovum and sperm also have the potential for becoming a human person and yet their loss at menstruation and ejaculation or by experimentation is accepted. It is true that the ovum and sperm are genetically unique but neither alone, even in the most favourable environment, will develop into a human person. They do not have this potential. The embryo, on the other hand, given the appropriate environment, will develop to the stage at which there would be general agreement that the status of a person be accorded to it. It must therefore be given special protection so that this potential can normally be fulfilled.

Experimentation

5. We would therefore support the creation of embryos with a view to their ultimate implantation in the uterus. The number created should be the optimum judged clinically to be necessary to secure implantation. More embryos should not be implanted than is clinically judged to be optimum solely because they have been created as this would both diminish the chance of their survival and expose the mother to the danger of multiple pregnancy. In the event of there being more embryos than is judged right to implant at any one time the remainder should either be frozen with a view to implantation at a later date or allowed to die. They should not be used for experimentation. Still less should embryos be deliberately created for the purpose of experimentation.

We therefore recommend that experimentation on the human embryo is not permitted.

Progress in treatment of infertility

6. A ban on experimentation will not halt progress in the treatment of infertility. Progress can still be made by animal and other experimentation and by the constant endeavour to improve the treatment procedure. Comparison with heart-transplantation makes this clear. Initial attempts were uniformly unsuccessful. Each attempt was however undertaken, with the hope of success; at no stage was a transplant undertaken with the intention the patient should not survive in order to gain knowledge as to how to improve the procedure. Continued therapeutic efforts backed by animal and other research

have produced steadily improving results. Likewise embryos should not be created with a view to their destruction in order to improve the results from *in vitro* fertilisation.

7. Infertility can be a heavy burden for an individual couple; it is right that efforts should be made to alleviate it. This does not however justify the use of any possible means. The advance of scientific knowledge is likewise of great value but again does not justify the use of any means. Because embryos have the potential to become human persons neither the relief of infertility nor the advance of knowledge justifies their deliberate destruction.

Consequences of permitting any experimentation

8. The ethical status of a procedure is determined by an analysis of the procedure itself. But when questions of public policy arise it is necessary also to look beyond the procedure to possible consequences. The proposal that the creation of embryos for research should be banned but that experiments on embryos created to relieve infertility which are no longer required for that purpose—so called "spare" embryos—be permitted, comes into this category. In our view experiments on "spare embryos" are wrong. But even if they were deemed right, the consequences of permitting them would be unacceptable. There would be a strong temptation for doctors to harvest more embryos than strictly required for the immediate therapeutic purpose in order to provide "spare embryos". "Spare" would become a euphemism.

9. Moreover as the number provided by this means would not meet the large demand foreseen by our colleagues the pressure for permission to create embryos specifically for research would grow. Likewise, limitations on the time and type of research would be eroded. Already voices are being raised for research to be permitted to a point beyond the fourteenth day after fertilisation recommended by this Inquiry. Similarly, if the use of embryos for testing of drugs, albeit under exceptional circumstances (12.8) were to be permitted, it would be difficult to maintain the limitation. Large numbers of new drugs are developed every year, many of which might be suitable for use by pregnant women. If a few were to be tested on embryos the demand for more to be screened in this way would inevitably grow. We conclude that experimentation on embryos

is not only unethical in principle but that the consequences of granting even limited permission for experimentation would be such as to lead inevitably to extensive use of embryos for this purpose.

10. *We therefore recommend that the embryo of the human species be afforded special protection in law.*

In order to achieve this legislation should be introduced to the effect that the unauthorised handling of a human embryo constitutes a criminal offence. Authorised handling should be under the control of a statutory licensing body which should have power to grant permission for the handling of embryos created with a view to implantation.

Madeline Carriline

John Marshall

Jean Walker

EXPRESSION OF DISSENT: C. USE OF HUMAN EMBRYOS IN RESEARCH

For the reasons set out in 11.25 to 11.27 inclusive, we dissent from the view that "research should be permitted on embryos brought into existence specifically for that purpose or coming into existence as a result of other research" (11.30).

Scott Baker

A O Dyson

N Edwards

Wendy Greengross

CONCLUSION

The Committee of Inquiry worked hard to produce its report, both in the time allotted, and, as we believe, with reasonable jargon-free clarity. That must, however, be for readers to judge. What I hope is that it will not have seemed, to those who have read it, a thoughtless or casual piece of work. We did our very best to consider all the arguments, and all the doctrines and expressions of feeling that came before us. We had, as well, to take account of our own very various opinions, which changed, in many cases, as we got deeper into the subject. But it is plainly not enough to plead that the report was the outcome of hard work and serious thought: so are many of the worst books in the world. The question has to be raised of its status. Will it, and should it, be taken as in any way authoritative? This in turn leads to the more general question, What is the standing of Committees of Inquiry such as ours?

In the first place, this was not, and could not be a committee of experts. Our task, as has been emphasised in the foregoing pages, was primarily to give advice to Ministers, based on moral judgments; and there is no such thing as a moral expert. Perhaps this point should be elaborated. Peter Singer and Deane Wells in their useful book *The Reproductive Revolution* (Oxford, 1984) argue that ethical committees set up to advise governments, if they are composed as ours was, with a general intention to include a fair number of different points of view, are bound to produce wishy-washy and feeble reports. The only way such a committee can produce the appearance of consensus out of pluralism is to give with one hand and take away with the other; to put one point of view and then immediately weigh against it another, until the issue is irrevocably fudged. They therefore argue that committees of inquiry into ethical issues should be made up of ethical experts. They realise that many people will find the idea of such an expert repugnant. But, they say, if reason and logical argument have any role to play in ethics it follows that the first requirement of the expert is to be able to reason well and detect errors in his own or other people's reasoning. In this sense at least there could be agreed experts. But there are other requirements too. An expert in ethics must understand the nature of ethics and the meaning of moral concepts. He may usefully have a fair knowledge of major ethical theories such as utilitarianism, or theories of rights or of justice. Finally an expert must be able to learn salient facts relevant to the issues to be settled.

Ethical experts so described do not sound very threatening. They do not sound like philosopher kings, who mysteriously know things that other people do not, or who have access to moral truths hidden from ordinary people. Indeed they sound like a collection of reasonably intelligent first-year philosophy students, following an introductory course in moral philosophy, and capable of benefitting from books and lectures. But of course it would be totally misleading to call such people experts. The only point of the expression is to suggest that their conclusions should be accepted without question. Other people, both Ministers who have sought their advice, and the public at large, must be prepared to say "the experts have decided that this or that is right; we are in no position to disagree." But no-one would say this kind of thing about the sort of "experts" Singer and Wells suggest. No-one would suppose for one moment that their statements carried any special authority. In matters of life and death, of birth and of the family, no-one is prepared to defer to judgments made on the basis of a superior ability in philosophy. For these are areas which are central to morality, and everyone has a right to judge for himself. Such issues indeed lie at the heart of society; everyone not only wants to make their own choices but are bound to do so. And this is why there cannot be moral experts. Everyone's conscience is his own. The Protestant tradition founded on such a belief runs very deep in this country.

In fact the question whether there are moral experts or not is something of a red herring. For even if all the members of the Inquiry had been professionally trained philosophers, even if they had been much more professional than Singer and Wells suggest, still they probably would not have agreed with one another. People feel strongly on the matters we had to discuss, and they feel in different ways, and this would have been true even if all members had been expert logicians, and had read the works of John Stuart Mill, and John Rawls. It cannot be too strongly emphasised that in questions of morality, though there may be better and worse judgments, there is no such thing as a correct judgment. That being so, no judgment can be imposed by one person on another as the only right or possible or proper judgment to make (even though each of us may feel that his judgment is manifestly best). This is why the notion of experts is not only out of place, but totally unacceptable.

If it is agreed, then, that there are no moral or ethical experts, what advantage do members of a committee such as ours have over other members of the public? Why should we have presumed to advise Ministers on matters with which everyone is equally concerned, and has an equal right to be thought competent? First, I suppose, it can be said that a committee, having been asked to make recommendations, has time to think about the issues. And this leads to the second and major advantage. They are in a position, through the civil service who form their secretariat, to discover as many facts as they can relevant to their enquiry, and to canvas as many opinions as they have time to listen to. All such Inquiries take written evidence, and most, including our own, seek oral evidence as well so that they can have the facts further explained or discuss the opinions in greater depth. People nearly always think that such committees take too little evidence, or pay too little attention to it; but I doubt whether this is so. They generally do the best possible in the allotted time. In this way, then, members of the committee, though at the beginning they may have been both ignorant and prejudiced, gradually acquaint themselves with the complexities of the facts and the differing moral values involved in the facts. So at the end though they are not moral experts, they are nevertheless in a position to base their judgments on knowledge. In the case of our Committee, for example, it was especially necessary that we should become familiar with the nature of early embryonic development, as far as is possible in the present state of scientific knowledge. We also had to distinguish various different forms of infertility treatment, and try as far as we could to ascertain their likely success rate. None of these things was particularly difficult to grasp, but some of them were quite difficult to find out, and in any case the ordinary public, and the "lay" members of the Committee were by no means familiar with the facts at the beginning. In these kinds of ways, then, though members of the Committee were not necessarily wiser than other people they became, and had a duty to become, better informed.

In one sense, then, the purpose of a committee such as ours is educational. For it must be the aim of the report that issues from it to share the knowledge which the committee has had time to gain, and to explain how their judgments flow from this knowledge. The explanation contained in the report, its educational content, is directed both to members of the public who are interested (and in our case that was practically all of society), and also to Members of Parliament who will have to consider the question of legislation.

It is often said that committees are set up only when Parliament wants to postpone legislation, to give themselves a breathing space. For it is very disagreeable to have to legislate on a controversial non-party matter which has wide public effects and the longer it can be put off the better. There is much truth in this. No government can look forward to legislating on matters in regard to which they know in advance that many voters will be outraged whatever they do. They may well wish to put off the evil hour. Nevertheless, on a more charitable view, it can be argued that if they did not establish a committee, Ministers would have to seek advice only from their own civil servants. Civil servants are often extremely cautious in the advice they give; and, much more important, they are necessarily secretive. No-one in the public at large knows who the particular civil servants are who proffer advice to Ministers. There is no guarantee that a variety of different views are considered, though doubtless this often happens. A committee of inquiry, on the other hand, though not exactly accountable to the public, is nevertheless far more open in its work, and a great deal less anonymous than the civil service. For this reason, if for no other, I believe that Ministers are fully justified in seeking advice in this way.

But, it may be said, why does a Minister not simply listen to the public? Why need he establish this go-between body, often seen as a cumbersome, expensive and inefficient extra, neither society itself, nor civil servants whose proper job it is to advise? The answer to this is largely implicit in what has already been said. An Inquiry is allowed time for fact-finding and reflection, and for sorting out the differences of opinion within society of which individuals may be unaware. But in addition there are obvious difficulties in the way of consulting "society as a whole". Who speaks for this creature? Is it the man on the Clapham omnibus, or those people who feel so strongly about a particular issue that they have formed themselves into a pressure group? Ministers would be a prey to pressures from all sides and would have the greatest difficulty in sorting out the sensible from the silly, the reasoned from the hysterical, the sane from the mad. I believe, in fact, that there may be an increasing number of issues where a go-between is necessary and desirable. People increasingly demand that legislation, when it comes, should be justified. When legislation follows a reasonably well-set-out report such justification is easy, the work has already been half done. Even if legislation does not take the form recommended by the Inquiry, still it is easier to explain the points of divergence if there is available a document which everyone can read and understand.

It has to be remembered that Ministers are not bound to follow advice they are given by committees of inquiry. The report is *only* advice. The recommendations begin to have force only if they seem sensible and persuasive to Ministers and their civil servants. There is indeed often disappointment on the part of members of committees who have worked hard and given the best advice they could, after what may seem endless consideration, only to see their report pigeon-holed forever. Equally, there must often be disappointment on the part of Ministers, who, understandably enough, may hope for a solution to a problem essentially insoluble. In the case of our Committee, for example, it was hoped, I now see, that the cool and reasonable voice of philosophy would reconcile the irreconcilable, and find a compromise where none can exist. There may even have been a secret belief that there is a right solution which could be proved right, if it were only found. But Ministers, like the rest of humanity, have to realise that in matters of morality this is not possible. Society may value things, genuinely and quite properly, which are incompatible with each other. Society as a whole values advances in science, especially in medicine; it values the possible new relief for the infertile, and the new hope of controlling crippling and disabling diseases. But the research upon which such advances depend seems to run counter to another highly prized value, the absolute sanctity of human life from its very earliest stage of development. There is, as the report itself demonstrates, no way of reconciling these values, in the sense of ensuring that everyone can be satisfied with a solution, that no-one will feel that too great a sacrifice is being asked. The majority of us held that the sanctity of human life in general can be upheld even if the very earliest and least developed embryos were used in research. But not everyone agrees. In the end it must be for Parliament to come to a decision about which value to place higher.

For there is no doubt that, whether or not the recommendations of the Inquiry are accepted in detail, there is agreement in society on one point: that legislation is necessary. Perhaps it would be true to say that our report had two main purposes, the first, as I have suggested above, broadly educational, the second practical, to help bring about changes in the law. At the educational level, we hoped among other things to cast some light on the new kinds of family that are becoming possible, and perhaps to influence the attitudes of the medical profession towards infertility treatment. As to the second purpose, we were conscious of an increasing sense of urgency that controls should be introduced where none exist, and that the law should be brought up to date, so that society may be protected from its real and very proper fear of a rudderless voyage into unknown and threatening seas.

APPENDIX
ORGANISATIONS SUBMITTING EVIDENCE

Those who gave oral evidence are marked with a star. Also listed are those individuals working in the field of human reproduction or on matters related to the issues examined by the Inquiry. In addition we received 695 letters and submissions from the public.

Action for Lesbian Parents
Agricultural Research Council
All Party Lords and Commons
    Family and Child Protection Group
Dr P J Armon MRCOG
Association for Spina Bifida and
    Hydrocephalus
Association of County Councils
Association of Directors of Social
    Services
*Association of District Committees
    for the Health and Personal Social
    Services, Northern Ireland
Association of Lawyers for the
    Defence of the Unborn
Association of Liberal Lawyers
Association of Nurse Administrators
Association to Combat Huntingtons
    Chorea

Baptist Union of Great Britain and
    Ireland
Baptist Union of Wales
Barnardo's
Bharatiya Vidya Bhavan—Institute of
    Indian Culture
Biosocial Society
Birmingham Maternity Hospital
Board for Social Responsibility of the
    General Synod of the Church of
    England
Board of Social Responsibility of the
    Church of Scotland
*Bourn Hall Clinic
*Dr P R Braude PhD MRCOG
British Agencies for Adoption and
    Fostering
British Association for the
    Advancement of Science
British Association of Social Workers

*British Council of Churches
British Evangelical Council
British Housewives League
British Industrial Biological Research
    Association
*British Medical Association
British Paediatric Association
British Pregnancy Advisory Service
British Toxicology Society
British Transplantation Society
Dr P D Bromwich MRCOG
Brook Advisory Centres

Campaign for Homosexual Equality
Campaign for Homosexual
    Equality—Tyneside Group
Campaign for Test Tube Freedom
Catholic Bishops Joint Committee on
    Bioethical Issues
Catholic Child Welfare Society
Catholic Marriage Advisory Council
Central Midwives Board for Scotland
Chancery Bar Association
*Chief Rabbi
CHILD
Christian Medical Fellowship
Church in Wales
Church of England Children's Society
Church of Ireland Adoption Society
    for Northern Ireland
Church of Ireland Armagh Diocesan
    Board of Social Responsibility
Clinical Medical Fellowship
Clinical Genetics Society
Clinical Theology Association
College of Arms
Community Health Councils:
    Barking, Havering and Brentwood
    Bassetlaw
    Chorley and South Ribble

Durham
East Cumbria
East Hertfordshire
Exeter and District
Gloucester and District
Grimsby
Isles of Scilly
Lancaster
Medway
Merton and Sutton
Newham
Nottingham
Peterborough
Richmond, Twickenham and
    Roehampton
Rochdale
Solihull
South Bedfordshire
South Warwickshire
West Berkshire
West Birmingham
Weston
Convention of Scottish Local
    Authorities
Council for Science and Society
Council for the Education and
    Training of Health Visitors
Council of Reform and Liberal
    Rabbis
Professor I Craft FRCS FRCOG
CRUX
D J Cusine, Senior Lecturer in Law,
    University of Aberdeen
Cystic Fibrosis Research Trust

Right Reverend Edward Daly, Bishop
    of Derry
Professor G David
Donors' Offspring
Down and Dromore and Connor
    Social Services Committee
Dumfries and Galloway Local Health
    Council
*Professor G R Dunstan

*Dr R G Edwards FRS PhD
Episcopal Church in Scotland
Ethico-Medical Committee of the
    Catholic Union of Great Britain and
    the Guild of Catholic Doctors

Faculty of Community Medicine of
    the Royal Colleges of Physicians of
    the UK
Family Care (Edinburgh)
Family Forum
Family Planning Association
Family Service Units
Family Welfare Association
Free Church Federal Council
Free Church of Scotland
Free Presbyterian Church of Scotland

General Nursing Council for England
    and Wales
Guild of Catholic Doctors: Dr P J
    Callaghan, Preston Branch
Guy's Hospital Medical School—
    Department of Community
    Medicine
Health Authorities (England and
    Wales):
    Brighton
    Crewe
    Dudley
    Durham
    Mid Glamorgan
    Rugby
    Shropshire
    South Birmingham
    Sunderland
    Torbay
    Walsall
Health and Social Services Boards
    (Northern Ireland):
    *Eastern
    Western
Health Boards (Scotland):
    Dumfries and Galloway
    Fife
    Highland
    Lanarkshire
    Lothian
    Tayside
Health Visitors Association
Rev Dr Walter Hedgcock
High Court of Justice—Family
    Division
Huntingdon Research Centre

*Incorporated Law Society of
    Northern Ireland

102

INFANT
Institute of Marital Studies
International Planned Parenthood
　Federation

Joint Board of Clinical Nursing
　Studies
Joint Coordinating Committee of the
　Medical Defence Organisations
Joint Standing Committee
　British Paediatric Society/Royal
　College of Obstetricians and
　Gynaecologists
Justices' Clerks' Society

I Kennedy, Professor of Medical Law
　and Ethics, Kings College, London
Knights of St Columbanus—
　Northern Area Committee

Lansdowne Baptist Church
Law Society
Law Society of Scotland
League of Jewish Women
LIFE

Dr Alexina McWhinnie
*Fr J Mahoney SJ
Magistrates Association—Inner
　Manchester Branch
Maternity Alliance
*Medical Research Council
Medical Women's Federation
Methodist Church Division of Social
　Responsibility
*Methodist Church in Ireland
*Professor G D Mitchell
Mothers' Union

National Abortion Campaign
National Association for the Childless
*National Association for the Childless
　(Northern Ireland)
National Association of Family
　Planning Doctors
National Association of Family
　Planning Nurses
National Association of Health
　Authorities in England and Wales
National Association of Maternal and
　Child Welfare

National Association of Ovulation
　Method Instructors
National Board of Catholic Women
National Childbirth Trust
National Childrens Homes
National Council for One Parent
　Families
National Council of Women in Great
　Britain
National Federation of Womens'
　Institutes
National Marriage Guidance Council
Nationwide Festival of Light
*Northern Ireland Council for Nurses
　and Midwives

Dr C D Ockleford

Panel of Assessors for District Nurse
　Training
Patients Association
Pharmaceutical Society of Great
　Britain
*Presbyterian Church of Ireland
Prebyterian Church of Wales

R W M Rees FRCS
Regional Health Authorities:
　East Anglian
　Durham
　Mersey
　Northern
　North Western
　North West Thames
　Oxford
　South East Thames
　South Western
　Trent
　West Midlands
Responsible Society
Rights of Women
Role of the Church Committee,
　Church of Ireland
Royal College of General Practitioners
Royal College of Midwives
Royal College of Nursing
*Royal College of Obstetricians and
　Gynaecologists
Royal College of Pathologists
Royal College of Physicians
Royal College of Physicians of
　Edinburgh

103

Royal College of Psychiatrists
Royal College of Surgeons
Royal College of Surgeons of
  Edinburgh
Royal Society
Royal Society for Mentally
  Handicapped Children and Adults

Salvation Army
Dr Bernard Sandler MD
Science Fiction Foundation
Scottish Council for Single Parents
Scottish Health Visitors Association
Senate of the Inns of Court and the
  Bar
*Dr R Snowden
Social Welfare Commission of the
  Catholic Bishops Conference
  (England and Wales)
Society for Reproductive and Infant
  Psychology
Society for the Protection of the
  Unborn Child
Soroptimist Club—Knutsford and
  District
Soroptimist International
Soroptimist International of Colwyn
  Bay and District
South London Islamic Mission
*P Steptoe FRCS FRCOG
St Georges Hospital Medical School
St Vincents Bioethics Centre
Study Commission on the Family
Professor E M Symonds MD FRCOG

Titus Trust
Trades Union Congress

*Ulster Obstetrical and Gynaecological
  Society
United Free Church of Scotland
United Kingdom Islamic Mission
United Kingdom Thalassaemia
  Society
Universities:
  Birmingham—Faculty of Medicine
    and Dentistry
  Bradford—Lecturer
  Cardiff—Department of
    Philosophy
  Dundee—Faculty of Medicine and
    Dentistry

Durham
—Faculty of Divinity
—Faculty of Law
—Department of Philosophy
Edinburgh
Glasgow
—Faculty of Medicine
  —Member of Department of
    Medical Genetics
Kent
Leeds
—Department of Medicine
—Department of Obstetrics and
  Gynaecology
—Department of Psychology
—Faculty of Law
Leicester—Department of
Anatomy
Liverpool
—Boards of Studies in
  Pharmacy, Psychology
—Faculty of Medicine
London
—Board of Studies in Pathology
—Board of Studies in
  Pharmacology
—Board of Studies in Psychology
—Chelsea College
—Department of Community
  Medicine
—Institute of Child Health
—Institute of Obstetrics and
  Gynaecology
—Kings College London
  Women in Science Group
—Queen Mary College
—St Mary's Hospital Medical
  School
—University College
  —Department of Hebrew
    and Jewish Studies
  —School of Medicine
  —Department of Obstetrics
    and Gynaecology
Loughborough—Technology
Manchester
—Department of Child Health
—Department of Obstetrics and
  Gynaecology
—Faculty of Law
Newcastle-upon-Tyne

Nottingham—Department of Obstetrics and Gynaecology

Oxford—Department of Social and Administrative Studies

Queens, Belfast
—Department of Surgery
—Faculty of Medicine

Reading

Sheffield—Department of Obstetrics and Gynaecology

Southampton
—Faculty of Law
—Faculty of Medicine

Surrey

York—Department of Biology

Voluntary Council for Handicapped Children

Welsh National School of Medicine

West Indian Standing Conference

Professor D J Weatherall FRS FRCP

Mr R W L Winston MRCOG

Women for Life

Women for Life on Earth

Women in Medicine

Women's National Commission

World Federation of Doctors Who Respect Human Life

Yorkshire Pro-Life Coordinating Committee

* Oral presentation made by representatives of the Working Party on Childlessness set up under the auspices of The Free Church Federal Council and The British Council of Churches.

INDEX

Double numbered references are to paragraph numbers in the text, roman numbering relates to the Introduction, arabic numbering to the Conclusion. XA refers to the First Expression of Dissent, XB refers to the Second Expression of Dissent, XC refers to the Third Expression of Dissent.